THE MAGIC OF RISING EARLY

THE MAGIC OF RISING EARLY

Authored By,

SACHIEN MANDAPPA

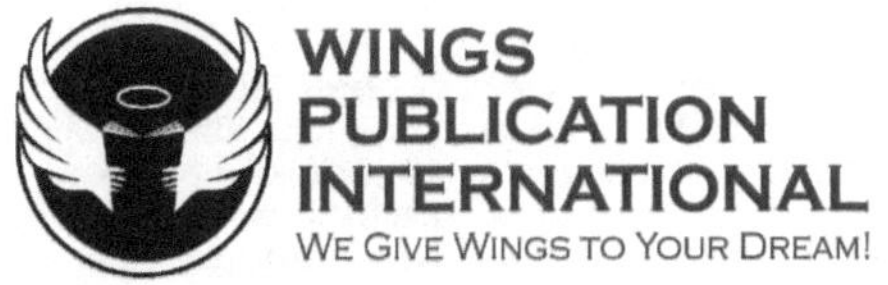

Disclaimer

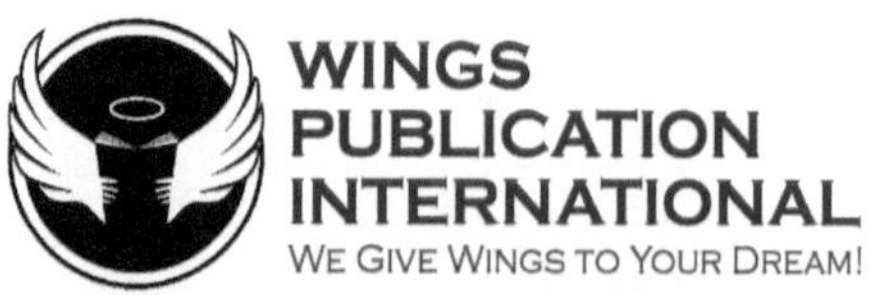

Registered Office- 907-Sneh Nagar, Sapna Sangeeta Road, Agrasen Square, Indore – 452001 (M.P.), India

Website: http://www.wingspublication.com

Email: mybook@wingspublication.com

First Published by WINGS PUBLICATION 2024

Copyright © SACHIEN MANDAPPA

Title : THE MAGIC OF RISING EARLY

Price : Rs. 1275/- | $ 15 | AED 55

All Rights Reserved.

ISBN : 978-93-6006-372-6

LIMITS OF LIABILITY/DISCLAIMER OF WARRANTY

Dedication

To my beloved wife, whose unwavering love and support have been my greatest strength.

To my son, who inspires me every day with his boundless curiosity and joy for life.

To my parents and my family for their constant encouragement and belief in me.

To all those who delve into these pages, may this book offer valuable guidance and serve as a wellspring of inspiration for their personal evolution and improvement in all aspects of life

Acknowledgement

I want to extend my deepest gratitude to Almighty God, the Universe, Mother Earth, and Planet Earth for their constant guidance and blessings. I am profoundly grateful to my parents and teachers, who laid the foundation for my growth and gave me the tools to be where I am today, enabling me to write this book.

A special thanks goes to those who played a crucial role in its creation: my loving wife, whose unwavering support and encouragement have been my greatest strength, and my dear son, whose inspiration fuels me every day. I also wish to thank my wonderful sisters and brother-in-law, who have stood by me through every stage of my life. Their love and support have been invaluable.

I am thankful to my dear friends and extended family, whose support and encouragement have brought warmth and strength to my life's journey. I am truly grateful to Dr. Kailash, Dr. Deepak, Ms. Varsha, and the entire Wings Publication Team; their dedication and guidance have been instrumental in shaping this book.

Lastly, I am deeply grateful to each reader who takes the time to journey through my words. This book was written to inspire and foster growth in your life, and I hope it ignites a spark of inspiration in you.

Thank you all for being part of this journey with me.

Preface

The pursuit of a life filled with balance, health, and fulfillment begins with the small yet powerful habits we cultivate each day. Imagine waking up each morning with a renewed sense of purpose, ready to embrace the day ahead. In this book, I invite you to explore transformative insights that not only turned my life around during a challenging time but can also empower you to rise above your struggles and discover a deeper sense of purpose.

Life often presents us with challenges that serve as powerful messages, urging us to reflect, grow, and find strength within ourselves. My journey was no exception; I found myself at a crossroads, feeling as though everything had gone off track. Yet, through simple daily practices, I discovered a path toward self-improvement and harmony with nature, my family, and, most importantly, myself. These insights are not just theoretical; they are rooted in real experiences that resonate deeply with anyone seeking positive change.

At the core of this book is the understanding of essential elements that shape our well-being—food, water, and our unique body constitution, or Prakriti. By aligning our dietary choices with ancient wisdom, we can nourish our bodies and minds effectively. Here, you will learn the art of mindful eating and hydration, allowing you to personalize your routines and nurture your health holistically.

Mornings hold immense transformative potential, offering a blank canvas to set the tone for the day. By developing intentional morning rituals that incorporate meditation, prayer, and mindful movement, you can infuse your life with energy and focus. Each chapter reveals how these simple yet impactful practices can create a foundation of purpose, guiding you through each day with intention.

In addition to morning routines, this book explores the power of daily rituals, including affirmations, gratitude, imagination, and visualization. These tools are not merely theoretical concepts; they are practical strategies that can help you manifest your dreams and aspirations. Complemented by physical activities such as exercise and intermittent fasting, these rituals foster a balanced and fulfilling lifestyle.

Evenings, too, play a crucial role in your journey. Discover how to cultivate a nourishing evening routine that prepares your body and mind for restful sleep, allowing you to greet each new day with renewed energy and enthusiasm. By integrating family routines, you'll not only strengthen bonds but also create a nurturing environment where everyone can thrive.

The book also delves into the principles of minimalism, illustrating how simplifying your life can lead to greater clarity and contentment. In a world filled with distractions, embracing a minimalist lifestyle allows you to focus on what truly matters, enhancing your overall well-being.

As you turn these pages, I encourage you to embark on your journey of daily success and personal growth. The small, consistent habits you develop—whether alone or with your family—have the power to transform your life. This book is your companion, guiding you toward becoming stronger, more centred, and deeply attuned to your highest values.

May the lessons within serve as a beacon on your path to discovering joy, balance, and fulfilment in your everyday existence. I invite you to take this step forward and unlock the potential for a life that reflects your aspirations.

About the book

Imagine a book that slowly unravels secrets to transforming your daily life—one small change at a time. With each chapter, you'll explore habits and routines that bring clarity, energy, and focus, all while hinting at a hidden key that ties them together. But there's a remarkable turn—a single practice that's quietly woven throughout, holding the power to elevate your mornings, sharpen your mind, and boost your well-being. What is this one habit that so many overlook? The deeper you go, the closer you'll get to uncovering it. And when you do, it might just change your life forever!

Who is this book for?

This book is designed for individuals seeking personal growth and improvement, including students, professionals, and anyone looking to enhance their daily routines. It's perfect for those feeling overwhelmed by life's demands and wanting to implement manageable changes for a better quality of life. Along with building better habits, this book will also help improve overall well-being, creating a balanced and healthier lifestyle.

Three benefits for readers:

1. **Clarity and Focus**: Learn how to prioritise what truly matters in your life.

2. **More Energy**: Discover simple changes that will boost your energy levels, making your days more vibrant.

3. **Better Well-being**: Uncover practices that enhance mental and emotional health, leading to a happier and more balanced life.

About the Author

Sachien Mandappa is an accomplished engineer who has been based in the UAE since 2005. Over the years, his professional journey has evolved, and today, he is a successful entrepreneur running his own business. Beyond his technical career, Sachien Mandappa is a passionate writer and a versatile drama artist, bringing stories to life through his unique creative lens. His love for storytelling began during his school and college days, where he actively directed and acted in numerous scripts, leaving a lasting impression on his peers. Although he has yet to publish his works in the public domain, his writing continues to be a profound medium of expression, reflecting his thoughts and experiences. With a blend of technical prowess and artistic flair, Sachien Mandappa brings a rare combination of insight and creativity to his endeavours, making his journey genuinely inspiring. He aims to share his passion, inspiring others along the way.

Contents

01

Beyond the Beginnings

Nothing is more responsible for the good old days than a bad memory.

\- Franklin Pierce Adams

Roots of Childhood

Growing up in a quaint village or a coffee estate surrounded by lush greenery and vibrant fields, I was enchanted by the warmth of the sun and the simple pleasures of rural life. Every morning, a lively group of us would walk miles to catch the bus that took us to our school in a neighbouring town. After school, I would return home to the comforting aroma of my mother's delicious home-cooked meals, signalling the start of our cherished evening supper routine. Rejuvenated after the meal, I would eagerly join my friends for lively games of cricket, played across the sprawling estate fields, savouring the joy of outdoor play until the sun sank below the horizon. As night approached, my father would come home after a long day, always offering advice and encouraging me to focus on my studies in the evening. By 8 PM, we would all sit down for dinner, and by 8:30 PM, we'd say our goodnights and head to bed, following our regular routine. Meanwhile, my mother would quietly plan for the next day, preparing breakfast and packing nutritious lunches for me and my two sisters to take to school.

Each morning, I woke up feeling refreshed, energised by the crowing rooster that roused my parents. While my mother managed our household with care, my father worked tirelessly on the coffee estate, which was the foundation of our livelihood. This routine remained consistent throughout the week, with Sunday being our treasured day of rest and relaxation. Sundays were a time to unwind and recharge for the week ahead, filled with the enjoyment of Doordarshan programs like *Rangoli*, regional movies, *Surabhi, and other TV programs*. These shows were a delightful escape, and the news broadcasts were informative, steering clear of negativity and positively impacting our lives.

Our days were filled with curiosity and creativity as we engaged in various indoor and outdoor activities. We especially loved bonding over games like Carom with our parents and sisters. Outdoors, we enjoyed a range of activities, from energetic sports to the serene art of pond fishing and crab-catching. We also found adventure in catching parrots and wandering through the peaceful coffee plantations on foot. The coffee was grown under the shade of Rosewood, Wild Fig, Jackfruit, and other native trees, creating a vibrant and diverse environment. During these walks, the scent of coffee bushes blended with the sweet fragrance of surrounding vegetation, accompanied by the soothing sounds of birds chirping and the occasional glimpse of wildlife. Being surrounded by nature, free from pollution, provided the perfect setting to rejuvenate both body and soul. Fresh air, calming sounds, and fragrant aromas contributed to a sense of deep tranquillity and connection with the natural world.

I discovered my love for cooking at a young age, and it always felt like something I was naturally meant to do. I don't recall anyone ever teaching me the art of cooking, but there is one vivid memory from when I was in fifth grade. My family had just purchased a new refrigerator and a kerosene stove that resembled a gas stove. One day, while my parents were out, I became eager to try the new stove. In my excitement, I accidentally poured kerosene into the tank while it was still on, causing a fire that quickly spread to one of the rooms, even slightly damaging the new refrigerator. Fortunately, some nearby labourers noticed the fire, rushed over with a wet gunny bag, and managed to put it out. I felt incredibly relieved and grateful for their help, but I knew I was in serious trouble when my parents returned. When it came time to explain what had happened, I struggled to find the right words. Thankfully, my father, who always had a soft spot for me, spared me from the scolding I rightfully deserved. This experience taught me a valuable lesson. I truly understood how dangerous fire could be and learned the importance of being cautious and responsible, even while following my passions.

I also fondly remember visiting our relatives, which always felt like a mini adventure. These trips were like a three-day picnic, filled with joy and excitement. Our journey would begin with a fun ride on a local bus. On the first day, we would enjoy a feast featuring the meat we brought. The second day was always special, as our relatives would prepare a delicious, spicy chicken dish made from a hen they had raised at home. We would spend the day laughing, sharing stories, and playing Antakshari, a lively game where we sang songs that started with the last letter of the previous song. Back then, we had plenty of time and countless topics to discuss without mobile phones or gadgets. Our conversations were rich and meaningful, full of shared information and messages. When it was time to leave, we would have a simple yet delicious breakfast of egg curry and rice roti before catching the local bus back home. The bus rides were entertaining, with fascinating people and beautiful landscapes to enjoy along the way. No matter what, the journey home always left us feeling refreshed, as though our spirits had been uplifted and our hearts filled with warmth from the time spent with loved ones.

The rainy season brought a mix of challenges and joy. While the constant downpours often disrupted our daily activities, they also offered moments of fun and togetherness. We would rush outside to play cricket whenever the rain paused, relishing the wet and muddy surroundings. Wearing a raincoat during middle school felt like an adventure in itself, as our excitement sometimes led to playful antics, leaving us wholly drenched despite our best efforts to stay dry. Surprisingly, this frequent exposure to rain seemed to make us stronger, helping us build resilience against the illnesses typically associated with damp weather.

The comforting sound of raindrops hitting the roof was a familiar backdrop, occasionally interrupted by the sight of small leaks that required makeshift buckets to catch the dripping water. These moments never failed to make us laugh, creating a sense of shared joy and bonding. As the rainy season drew to a close, we eagerly anticipated the harvest festival. The tantalising aromas of bamboo shoot curry, tapioca leaf curry, and taro leaf dishes filled the air, whetting our appetites and building excitement for the delicious meals.

During the Kakkada or Ashada season, typically occurring in July or August, the air is filled with the mouth-watering aroma of homemade chicken curry alongside Coorg's signature dishes like Pandi Curry (a pork delicacy) and Kadambutte (steamed rice balls). Many families cherish these traditional meals in Coorg. A unique aspect of the Kakkada season is the preparation of a special herb-based dish called Aati Payasa (payasam) on the 18th day, the last day of kakkada. Local tradition holds that the medicinal properties of this herb are at their peak on the 18th day of Kakkada, marking the season's end, making it particularly beneficial when consumed on that day. However, for many of us, the true joy of indulging in payasam wasn't just about its delightful taste or health benefits; it was more about the playful thrill of seeing our urine turn a surprising shade of red! This curious and amusing side effect was caused by the natural colour change of the herbs during cooking. It became a light-hearted source of laughter and wonder, adding an unexpected twist to our culinary experience and turning each bowl of payasam into a playful adventure.

This cherished tradition and the enticing seasonal aromas added to the rich tapestry of flavours and experiences that Kakkada brought. In earlier times, we were lucky to witness clear seasonal changes—winter, spring, summer, pre-winter, autumn, and monsoon—arriving with precision, which filled us with pride in nature's rhythm. Each season had its own distinct charm and sense of anticipation, deepening our appreciation of life in Coorg. A local poet captured the very essence of these changing seasons through his eloquent verses, which painted vivid pictures of the valley's beauty. His lyrical expressions left a lasting impression on us during our visits, helping us appreciate the harmony between nature and the cycle of time even more profoundly.

Life on a coffee estate is deeply rooted in rich traditions and daily routines, with one of the most important events being the annual pooja. This sacred ceremony unites the entire community in the worship of the Gods and Goddesses believed to safeguard the plantation. During the pooja, residents offer goats and hens as sacrifices to Goddess Mariamma and other deities. Following the ritual sacrifice, the meat is shared among the residents, with a portion sold to raise funds. These funds are then used to organise a grand feast for the whole community, fostering a sense of unity and celebration.

The feast is a joyful occasion where relatives are warmly invited, strengthening familial bonds and bringing everyone closer together. It serves as both a celebration of religious devotion and an expression of community spirit, with food, laughter, and shared experiences creating lasting memories for all who participate.

In addition to the estate poojas, special rituals are conducted in the **Devara Kaadu**, sacred forests that serve as holy grounds for the local deities. Throughout Coorg, numerous such sacred groves exist, varying in size and significance. Some are vast, resembling small forests, while others are more modest in scale. These sacred spaces hold deep cultural and spiritual significance for the community, further enriching life on the coffee estate.

I have fond memories of the coffee harvesting season, which typically coincides with the February monsoon. Watching the coffee plants in full bloom and inhaling their delightful fragrance during February and March was always a captivating experience. Our summer holidays were often spent birdwatching, a favourite pastime during the pruning of the coffee trees. We would spot various birds, including woodpeckers, parrots, wood pigeons, and bulbuls, making each season special in its own way.

Above all, my mother's incredible ability to manage our household and care for our family single-handedly was a constant source of inspiration. Her dedication made every season even more memorable for us. One of my favourite memories is our family outings, especially our trips to the local movie theatre. I vividly recall one Sunday evening when we couldn't find a bus to take us home. Instead of being upset, my parents spontaneously decided to take me to watch a Kannada movie called *Premaloka*. Although I was too young to fully grasp the romantic storyline, the beautiful songs from the film left a lasting impression on me. It turned out to be a delightful surprise! After the movie, we took an auto-rickshaw home, happily reminiscing about our wonderful evening together.

I also treasure the times we spent listening to the large radio in our family home, where my father would tune in to various programs. After my elder sister got married, my brother-in-law would visit us every weekend. He would arrive on Saturday evenings and spend all of Sunday relaxing. Although we now live in a more technologically advanced era, we relied on manual methods for most tasks back then. Our lives were filled with experiences that taught us valuable lessons, and we took pleasure in simple activities that provided essential information. People were deeply connected to their social circles and followed a structured routine, starting their days early and enjoying coffee while reading the morning newspapers. They had excellent language skills, sharp eyesight, and a sense of harmony between their minds, bodies, and emotions.

Our neighbours, especially the women, would rise early to create intricate rangoli designs on their spotless floors. They managed most household chores without the help of hired maids, keeping them mentally and physically fit. People were fully engaged in their daily routines, utilising their bodies, minds, and emotions. Most individuals, especially housewives, dedicated themselves wholeheartedly to family tasks, providing love, care, and full involvement in family life.

Schoolyard Memories

Every festival, occasion, and event was celebrated with immense enthusiasm and joy. We were always eager to understand the cultural significance behind each celebration, embracing their meaning with pride. In the charming villages, lively folk games filled the air near the paddy fields, with ponds echoing with laughter and excitement. Dasara sports were not just events; they were meticulously planned and prepared with passion. Participants dedicated months to rigorous training, infusing the competition with energy and spirit.

Likewise, our school events were marked by a strong sense of camaraderie among classmates and schoolmates. Various activities—ranging from singing and fashion shows to quizzes, mono-acting, mimicry, handwriting competitions, flower arrangements, essay writing, and indoor and outdoor sports—brought out the best in each of us. These events allowed us to showcase our talents and creativity. Most of us scripted and practised for these activities independently, with minimal help from our parents. The climax was always the prize distribution, where students could win up to four prizes. I vividly recall the thrill of being honoured with five awards, only to have one taken back later. I owe a special thanks to my sisters, whose skills and talents contributed to some of my victories.

One particular memory from my school days stands out. In the 6th standard, I had scripted and participated in a play in Malayalam—a language my classmates barely understood but one I had picked up. We mainly communicated in English and Kannada, with a bit of Hindi. Around this time, I discovered my love for writing and began crafting articles and scripts. This newfound passion quickly became a cherished hobby. As I progressed through my academic journey, my involvement in scriptwriting intensified, becoming a significant part of my life by the time I reached the 8th, 9th, and 10th standards. Along with writing, I developed a passion for singing, especially in Kannada, Hindi, and Tamil. I have fond memories of performing movie songs, folk tunes, and poems—each performance holds a special place in my heart, evoking nostalgic emotions to this day.

College Days: Living the Experience

After completing my 10th standard, I left my hometown to pursue Pre-University (PU) studies. This marked the beginning of my hostel life, away from the comforting presence of my parents and the familiar surroundings of home. Having grown up in a place with a pleasantly moderate climate, I was unprepared for the extreme heat of my new environment.Everything around me changed dramatically—from the climate and food to the location and the company of friends in this entirely new setting. Immersing myself in the local way of life allowed me to experience diverse cultures, traditions, and languages firsthand. It's fascinating how India, much like a subcontinent, offers a rich tapestry of cultures, cuisines, and dialects, with noticeable changes every 100 kilometres. What struck me most was the variety in food every 100 miles, whether it was street food, home-cooked meals, village fare, tribal dishes, or the unique local country food, each adding a distinct flavour to the journey.

Hostel life imparted several valuable lessons, particularly the importance of punctuality. The fixed breakfast, lunch, and dinner timings instilled a sense of order in my daily routine. I had set wake-up times and designated slots for using the bathroom, and ensuring I arrived at my college classes on time was crucial. While I enjoyed playful mischief with friends and roommates during holidays and breaks, hostel life helped me develop a more disciplined lifestyle. I learned to manage my time efficiently and adapt to the new environment, which played a pivotal role in shaping my character and preparing me for future challenges.

Engineering Days

As an engineering student, I found myself living independently, without the structured routine that had been so central to my childhood. Back then, I would be fast asleep by 8:30 PM, but those four years of college life were vastly different. I often stayed up late into the night, sometimes even until the early morning, socialising with friends or attending parties. Without a set schedule or clear goals, I drifted through my studies, a sharp contrast to the disciplined upbringing I had known.

Looking back, I now realise the significance of having a daily routine and living a disciplined life. Each phase of my journey— from my early years to college and now in my professional and family life—has imparted valuable lessons. Many of us experience similar transitions, facing both success and challenges along the way. The real test, however, lies in how we handle our current circumstances and overcome internal and external hurdles. While everyone has the freedom to shape their own path, true success comes from staying committed to it with dedication, determination, and devotion, ultimately leading to a disciplined and fulfilling life.

During those days, before the era of gadgets, emails, and social media, writing was one of the main hobbies we cultivated. My father had a love for sending greeting cards on special occasions, and I embraced this tradition, sending cards to friends and relatives. While away from my parents, with limited access to landline phones, letters became our primary means of communication. Writing letters creatively and sharing news and moments became a cherished practice for me. I typically wrote one or two letters a month to my parents and sisters, and I always looked forward to their responses, filled with excitement and curiosity until their letters finally arrived.

When I read my mother's letters, I could visualise her face, feeling an intimate connection with her through the words. My passion for writing also sparked a love for collecting stamps and greeting cards, adding another dimension to my hobbies. I developed a keen interest in writing scripts during this period as well. Reading and writing became central to my daily routine, and I frequently visited the college library, which became an invaluable resource. There, I discovered new books, titles, and authors, fuelling my intellectual curiosity and serving as my primary source of knowledge during those formative years.

Professional Life

Since 2005, I have been living in the UAE, adopting a professional and responsible lifestyle with my wife and son. My time here has been enriched with meaningful experiences, and the fast-paced nature of city life has imparted its fair share of both positive and challenging lessons. I hold my life in high regard and am deeply grateful for the opportunities and experiences I have gained in the United Arab Emirates.

My parents, sisters, and brothers-in-law have always been my pillars of strength, guiding me through my education and helping me build a fulfilling life in the UAE. My parents' unwavering dedication and hard work set the foundation for my character, while my sisters provided constant encouragement during difficult times. Both of my brothers-in-law have enriched our family with their perspectives, further strengthening our bond. I also draw immense strength from my wife's unconditional love and support, which has created a nurturing and joyful environment for our family. My son's laughter and curiosity fill our lives with happiness, reminding me of life's simple joys. The love and connection I share with my extended family and friends continue to reinforce my sense of purpose and belonging.

Nature played a profound role in shaping my values and imparting key life lessons, offering a buffer from the world's harsher realities. Embracing a child's perspective and experiencing the marvels of growth and discovery were truly rewarding. Every moment seemed significant, filled with curiosity, happiness, and wonder. I often find myself reminiscing about those cherished times, which continue to warm my heart. The simplicity of days spent exploring the natural world and living without worry is something I deeply treasure.

Nostalgic Reflections

The belief that "the past was better" is known as nostalgia or nostalgic bias. This psychological tendency is common and has led to many discussions. Some people support this belief, while others present counterarguments. Let's explore both sides.

Supporting Arguments for "The Past Was Better"

Many people view the past through a lens of simplicity, recalling a time without modern technology, social media, and the fast-paced lifestyles we have today. This earlier period is often seen as more peaceful and connected, characterised by close-knit communities where families spent quality time together.

Creativity thrived in the past as people engaged in hands-on activities, crafting, and imaginative play. Children found joy in simple games and storytelling, fostering a sense of happiness that often felt genuine and untainted. In those days, curiosity was nurtured through exploration and nature, encouraging children to discover the world around them without the distractions of screens.

Honesty and discipline were commonly valued traits, with individuals often adhering to traditional norms and ethical standards. These qualities helped maintain strong community bonds, ensuring respect for elders and a sense of responsibility among younger generations. Life's surprises came in the form of spontaneous adventures, from discovering a hidden path in the woods to sharing stories around a campfire, making every moment feel special.

In the past, communication often happened through letters and greeting cards, which added a personal touch to relationships. Receiving a handwritten letter or a special card felt meaningful and created lasting memories. People looked forward to these messages, which deepened their connections.

Supporters of the idea that the past was better often reminisce about a time when life felt less hurried and work-life balance seemed easier to manage. They believe that people enjoy longer, healthier lives in harmony with nature, leading to a more idyllic existence. Psychological studies suggest that people tend to remember positive experiences more vividly than negative ones. This selective recall reinforces the belief that the past was better. We often filter out less pleasant memories, allowing the positive ones to dominate our thoughts.

Arguments Against "The Past Was Better"

However, it's crucial to recognise that many societies faced significant social injustices throughout history. Issues such as racial discrimination, gender inequality, and limited opportunities for marginalised groups were common. While the past had its challenges, modern technology has greatly improved various aspects of our lives.

For instance, advances in healthcare have allowed for more accurate diagnoses and effective treatments for many illnesses. Communication technology has changed how we connect, making it easier to stay in touch and access information. Innovations like electric vehicles and improvements in public transportation have made travel more convenient and contributed to a healthier environment.

At present, creativity has evolved, with technology offering new platforms for artistic expression. Social media allows for sharing ideas and connecting with others worldwide, fostering collaboration and innovation. However, the rapid pace of life can sometimes overshadow opportunities for deep, meaningful connections.

While happiness in the past often came from simple pleasures, today's world offers diverse experiences and the chance to pursue passions. Individuals can engage in various activities, from travel to hobbies, but the pressure of modern life can also lead to stress and burnout.

Moreover, today's digital tools and online resources have made learning more accessible, helping create a more informed society. Modern economies have improved living standards and granted access to goods that were once considered luxuries. Despite the imperfections of contemporary society, we have made significant strides in promoting inclusivity and social justice. Global poverty rates have declined, and access to education and job opportunities has improved significantly. Recent advancements in medical science have extended human life expectancy and enhanced the overall quality of life. Illnesses that were once fatal can now be effectively treated, improving countless individuals' health outcomes.

Psychological studies indicate that the belief that "the past was better" is often influenced by selective memory and emotional bias. People focus on the positive aspects of their experiences. However, when analysed objectively, it becomes clear that substantial advancements in health, technology, and social justice have made many aspects of modern life preferable to those of the past.

The Contrast Between Past and Present

While the past may appear simpler and more connected, it also had challenges that we often overlook when viewed through a nostalgic lens. For example, expressions of love and affection were primarily conveyed through personal gestures and actions. In contrast, today's society often commodifies love and affection, exchanging them for monetary value. Despite this shift, it is essential to remember that every journey has a beginning and an end. What truly matters is our ability to make meaningful contributions that leave a lasting impact on the lives of others.

Ultimately, individuals possess the freedom to make their own choices based on personal preferences and experiences. Whether one prefers the simplicity of the past or the convenience of modern life is a matter of personal perspective. Each person's journey is unique, shaped by their reflections on both the past and present.

02

The Foundations of Life: Food, Prakriti, Water and Ancient Insights

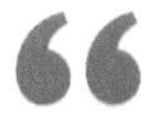

One key to success is to have lunch at the time of day most people have breakfast.

- Robert Brault

Food

The Role of Food in Human Life

Food is crucial for living beings as it provides the necessary energy and essential nutrients for physical and cognitive development, the maintenance of life processes, and the stimulation of growth. It serves as a complex amalgamation of chemical compounds, each with its own distinct role in the body's functioning. Furthermore, food is pivotal in promoting and sustaining overall health and preventing various diseases and health conditions.

Food as a Cultural Connector

Throughout human civilisation, food has played a significant role in shaping cultural traditions and fostering a sense of community. Culinary practices and rituals related to sustenance form the bedrock of identity and connection across the world's diverse cultures. The timing of meals, a vital aspect of these practices, has varied widely, reflecting the rich tapestry of human experiences and historical evolution. As a result of industrialisation and globalisation, there has been a move towards a more standardised approach to meal timing, with the traditional three-meal structure of breakfast, lunch, and dinner gaining importance. Even within this framework, there is significant diversity in the timing of meals. The recent upheavals brought about by the pandemic, such as periods of self-isolation, changes in working hours and patterns, and shifts in professional lifestyles, have further tested these traditions, leading to a more erratic and unpredictable eating pattern. However, the role of food in fostering community remains a constant, binding us together in a larger cultural narrative.

The Evolution of Meal Patterns

The practice of eating three meals a day – breakfast, lunch, and dinner – evolved gradually over centuries, influenced by changes in agriculture, societal norms, and cultural practices. Before settled agricultural societies, people ate whenever food was available through foraging or hunting. With the advent of the Agricultural Revolution, around 10,000 BCE, communities became more sedentary, and food production stabilised. As a result, people began to eat meals at more regular times of the day, often timed with their work schedules and the natural cycles of daylight. In these early farming societies, meals were typically communal and aligned with daily tasks. The main meal was usually consumed after labour-intensive activities like farming. As agricultural practices progressed, so did the structure of eating, with specific times for meals emerging based on work hours and natural light.

Historical Perspectives on Meals

Breakfast became a more distinct meal in medieval Europe, especially for the upper classes. While common folk often ate light, simple meals such as bread, cheese, or porridge in the morning, the nobility began to embrace larger, more elaborate breakfasts by the 16th century. This shift was partly due to changing societal expectations and the availability of more luxurious foods. Breakfast was considered a way to replenish energy after a night's sleep and prepare for the day's work or leisure.

Lunch has a more varied history compared to breakfast and dinner. In medieval times, a midday meal was common, particularly for manual labourers who needed sustenance to continue working through the day. As societies industrialised in the late 18th and 19th centuries, especially during the Industrial Revolution, workers required a light, portable meal that could be eaten quickly during breaks. This need gave rise to the modern concept of lunch, which was usually a simple meal that could be consumed easily and speedily, fitting into the fast-paced schedules of urban workers. By the mid-19th century, lunch was commonly eaten between 12 PM and 2 PM, aligning with the schedules of factory and office workers.

Dinner has historically been the day's main meal, but its timing and significance have varied. In early medieval times, dinner was often eaten in the early afternoon. However, as the upper classes gained influence, particularly in the 18th century, dinner was served later in the day, often between 6 PM and 8 PM. This shift was due to a combination of longer working hours, greater availability of leisure time, and technological advancements such as gas and electric lighting, which allowed people to dine after dark.

The Structure of Modern Meals

During the 19th and 20th centuries, due to social and cultural influences, meal patterns underwent significant formalisation, especially within the middle and upper classes. In the Victorian era, meal patterns became highly structured, reflecting the era's focus on etiquette and social class. Breakfast was served around 8–9 AM, often a substantial meal with items like eggs, meats, and tea. Lunch, or "luncheon," emerged as a lighter midday meal, typically eaten between 1–2 PM. Dinner, the main meal, was held later in the evening, usually between 6–8 PM, and was a formal affair for the upper classes, often with multiple courses. Supper, a lighter meal, was sometimes taken before bed. This structured pattern reinforced social status and formal dining rituals.

In today's modern society, the traditional meal schedule consisting of breakfast, lunch, and dinner continues to be widely observed, albeit with cultural nuances. Breakfast is often considered essential for providing the energy needed to start the day, while lunch offers a welcome respite during the demands of work or school. The evening meal, usually dinner, has evolved into a time for families to come together and engage in social interaction. The specific timing of these meals can vary significantly depending on individual lifestyle choices, cultural traditions, and personal preferences. However, the overarching framework of three distinct meals has become the norm in many communities worldwide.

Embracing Natural Eating Patterns

The transition from irregular eating patterns in ancient societies to the more organised three-meal structure seen in modern times results from a complex interplay of cultural, economic, and technological shifts throughout history. The historical and cultural development of breakfast, lunch, and dinner is a prime example of the intricate relationship between human behaviour and societal progress. These designated mealtimes have been shaped by agricultural practices, social frameworks, and evolving lifestyles, adapting over time to synchronise with the demands and rhythms of daily life.

In today's society, although there may be variations in specifics, the notion of three daily meals remains a cornerstone of many cultures, signifying tradition and the intricacies of contemporary existence. The evolution towards the structured three-meal system we are familiar with today underscores the profound interconnectedness of cultural traditions, economic progress (such as advancements in agriculture and industrialisation), and technological innovations (such as the development of lighting and refrigeration). Over time, these factors have reshaped how people eat, influencing the timing and content of meals and transitioning from sporadic, necessity-based eating to a more regular breakfast, lunch, and dinner schedule.

Jain Dietary Practices

The dietary customs of the Jain tradition are deeply rooted in the principle of ahimsa, which translates to non-violence and is meticulously crafted to minimise harm to all living beings. One significant practice involves consuming the final meal of the day before sunset. This practice is based on the belief that eating after dark might inadvertently harm minuscule organisms that are not visible in reduced light. By consuming their last meal before sunset, Jains aim to minimise this risk and remain true to their commitment to non-violence. While eating before sunset is crucial for Jains, the degree of adherence may vary based on individual beliefs and practices. The dietary restrictions within Jainism are exceptionally stringent, encompassing vegetarianism and the avoidance of root vegetables to prevent harm to plants and microorganisms.

Furthermore, the early evening meal aligns with the Jains' spiritual discipline and ascetic practices, providing an opportunity for proper digestion and reflection before sleep. This tradition exemplifies a profound respect for all forms of life and reinforces their lifestyle choices, including strict vegetarianism and the avoidance of root vegetables, all aimed at minimising harm to the environment and living beings.

The Benefits of Eating with the Natural Rhythm

In addition to these spiritual beliefs, modern scientific research supports this ancient practice, emphasising the benefits of early dining for improved digestion, metabolism, and overall health. Embracing the natural eating patterns of our ancestors, which designate specific times for breakfast, lunch, and dinner, is considered optimal. While contemporary life may require some adjustments to these traditional timings, striving to adhere to them as closely as possible can still provide significant health benefits.

Observing the natural world, we can see that animals and birds typically eat during the day and sleep at night, exhibiting robust health. They usually start eating at sunrise and avoid consuming food one hour before or after sunset. For humans, the recommended time for breakfast is 1-2 hours after sunrise, around 6 AM–8 AM. Lunch is best consumed between 12 Noon and 2 PM, and dinner is ideally eaten 1 hour before sunset, around 5 PM–6 PM. Embracing a daily 12- to 14-hour window of allowing the body to repair and recoup, known as "Intermittent Fasting," from 8:00 PM to 8:00 AM, can offer many benefits.

Optimal Meal Timing

Given our daily commitments, it is optimal to select the time as follows:

Breakfast: 06:00 AM—08:00 AM

It is recommended to have breakfast within one to two hours of waking up or roughly one to two hours after sunrise. This timing helps jumpstart your metabolism and provides the essential energy needed to begin your day. However, some individuals may prefer to wait a bit longer and enjoy their breakfast in the mid-morning instead. The ideal time is between 6:00 AM and 8:00 AM.

Lunch: 12:00 Noon—02:00 PM

Usually, between 12:00 noon and 2:00 PM, taking a midday break and refuelling your body by having lunch is recommended. This can help you replenish your energy levels and stay focused for the rest of the day. However, it is essential to consider individual preferences and schedules, as some people may find it more suitable to have lunch earlier or later based on their specific needs and hunger levels.

Dinner: 06:00 PM—08:00 PM

Dinner should ideally be eaten before sunset, which is typically between 6:00 PM and 8:00 PM. Having an early dinner allows your body to digest the food before sleep and prevents sleep disturbances related to heavy meals. This timing can also enhance overall well-being and facilitate better sleep.

Intermittent Fasting: 08:00 PM—08:00 AM

To maximise health benefits, allow your body to rest and rejuvenate during nighttime hours. Following an intermittent fasting schedule, such as having your last meal at 8:00 PM and breaking the fast at 8:00 AM the next day, aligns with natural biological rhythms and can lead to improved metabolic health.

Prakriti

Prakriti: The Foundation of Ayurvedic Nutrition

According to Ayurveda, food is classified as an Earth Element, and it is essential to consume food that aligns with our individual **Prakriti,** or constitution. This fundamental concept has gained extensive attention from modern medical sciences. To fully grasp the notion of Prakriti, it is vital to understand the human body's composition as described in Ayurveda. Adhering to one's Prakriti can yield remarkable results, often evoking a sense of almost magical influence on overall well-being.

The Interplay of Structure and Function

Ayurveda emphasises the intricate relationship between structure and function within the human body. It is proposed that as bodily functions, particularly digestion, become optimised, there is a corresponding improvement in the overall physical form. This suggests that when digestion processes operate efficiently, the body can create the precise amount of tissue required. This concept underscores that the body's structure is closely linked to its internal functional dynamics. Furthermore, Ayurveda posits that three distinct functional environments govern the various functions of the human body, each playing a unique role within its systems.

The First Functional Environment: Vata

The First Functional Environment in Ayurveda is responsible for controlling all types of movements, both gross and subtle. Gross movements include walking, gesturing, and speaking, while subtle movements encompass blood flow, nerve impulses, and intestinal contractions. These movements are profoundly influenced by a factor known as **Vata.**

Individuals with a Vata Prakriti exhibit qualities of dryness, lightness, coldness, and airiness. To maintain balance and prevent Vata imbalances, it is recommended that they consume foods with certain qualities, such as sweet foods like root vegetables, grains, and dairy. Moist foods like soups and stews, as well as those cooked with healthy oils, are beneficial. Consuming warm foods instead of raw or cold foods is also advised, as this helps counteract the natural dryness and coldness of Vata. Conversely, individuals should avoid cold foods, such as salads and iced drinks, as well as dry foods, like crackers and light snacks, which can exacerbate Vata imbalances and lead to issues like anxiety and digestive irregularities.

The Second Functional Environment: Pitta

The Second Functional Environment pertains to all processes related to transformation within the body, including digestion, metabolism, and energy conversion. Whenever there is a change in the form of substances within the body or an exchange of energy, it is attributed to this environment, primarily influenced by **Pitta.**

Individuals with a Pitta Prakriti possess a fiery and intense nature. They benefit from consuming foods with specific qualities, such as bitterness (found in leafy greens, turmeric, and bitter vegetables), light steaming of vegetables, and moderate warmth (avoiding excessively hot foods). These qualities aid in cooling and soothing the natural heat of Pitta, helping to prevent overheating, inflammation, and irritability. Foods that should be minimised include excessively hot, sour, and spicy dishes, as these can exacerbate Pitta's heat and lead to conditions such as acid reflux and skin rashes.

The Third Functional Environment: Kapha

The Third Functional Environment, known as **Kapha,** is

responsible for structure and storage within the body. This environment governs stability, lubrication, and support of bodily tissues. Individuals with a Kapha Prakriti tend to be heavy, moist, and slow, benefiting from a diet rich in specific food types. Recommended foods include bitter foods such as leafy greens and turmeric, dry-roasted items like grains and legumes, and warm, cooked meals to stimulate digestion and promote lightness.

Foods to avoid for those with a Kapha constitution include sweet items, cold foods like ice cream and raw vegetables, and dairy products. Consumption of these foods can exacerbate Kapha's natural heaviness and moisture, potentially leading to stagnation and sluggishness. Therefore, incorporating light, dry, and warm foods is essential for maintaining balance.

The Triad of Health: Vata, Pitta, and Kapha

KAPHA represents the physical foundation supporting VATA and PITTA functions in the human body. These three elements are vital for maintaining overall health and well-being, and understanding one's specific body type is crucial for optimal health and nutrition.

A successful diet should seamlessly integrate into one's lifestyle, making healthy eating feel like second nature. It's not just about consuming nutritious food but also about choosing foods suited to one's unique constitution. Some foods may not be compatible with your body, even if they are generally considered healthy. Prioritising easily digestible foods tailored to your Prakriti is recommended for optimal health.

A Holistic Perspective on Health

"Our health is not just the absence of illness, but a complete state of well-being encompassing mental, physical, emotional, and spiritual aspects. We often prioritise physical health while neglecting mental, emotional, and spiritual wellness. Instead of striving for perfection, we should focus on progress in all areas. Adopting best practices and constantly seeking improvement in every aspect of our health is essential."

Water

Hydration and Well-being

Maintaining proper hydration is essential for overall bodily function and well-being. Individuals should aim to consume adequate fluids, especially water, to satisfy their thirst. To minimise the likelihood of disrupting sleep with frequent trips to the bathroom, it is advisable to avoid consuming water at least two hours before bedtime. The U.S. National Academies of Sciences, Engineering, and Medicine recommends an average daily fluid intake of about 3.7 litres (125 ounces) for men and about 2.7 litres (91 ounces) for women in temperate climates. This intake includes fluids from water, other beverages, and food, with approximately 20% of the daily fluid intake coming from food and 80% from drinks.

Factors Influencing Water Intake

However, physical activity, climate, and overall health can

influence these requirements. Many health professionals recommend drinking between 250ml and 500ml of water in the morning or before meals. The commonly suggested guideline of "8 glasses of water a day" can be estimated at approximately 2 litres, assuming each glass contains around 250ml. Adequate hydration maximises physical performance, particularly during intense exercise. Additionally, staying well-hydrated helps sustain mental energy levels, prevent headaches, alleviate constipation, reduce the risk of kidney stones, aid in weight management, and promote healthy, radiant skin, among other benefits.

Adjusting Fluid Intake Based on Lifestyle

It is vital to keep your body hydrated by regularly consuming fluids, especially water, to satisfy your thirst. While some individuals may find that consuming less than eight glasses of water daily is adequate, others may require more. Your total fluid intake may need to be adjusted based on various factors, some of which are as follows:

1. Physical Activity: Engaging in physical activities that cause sweating necessitates increasing water consumption to replenish lost fluids. It's crucial to drink water before, during, and after exercising.

2. Climate Conditions: Hot or humid weather conditions can increase sweating, requiring additional fluid intake to prevent dehydration. This is particularly important in regions with high temperatures or at high altitudes.

3. Health Issues: Certain health issues, such as fever, vomiting, or diarrhoea, can result in bodily fluid loss. Increasing water intake or following a doctor's recommendation to consume oral rehydration solutions is essential. Conditions like bladder infections and urinary tract stones may also require heightened fluid intake.

4. Pregnancy and Breastfeeding: Pregnant or breastfeeding individuals may need additional fluids to ensure proper hydration for themselves and their infants.

You can effectively maintain optimal hydration levels by considering these factors and adjusting your fluid intake.

Alternative Sources of Hydration

When it comes to maintaining proper hydration, it's essential to remember that water isn't the sole source of fluids for your body. In addition to drinking water, you can also fulfil your body's hydration needs by consuming certain foods. Various fruits and vegetables, such as watermelon, cucumbers, and spinach, are packed with high water content, significantly keeping you hydrated. Apart from these, beverages like milk, juice, and herbal teas are predominantly made up of water and can contribute to your overall fluid intake. Interestingly, even caffeinated drinks like coffee and soda can add to your daily hydration. However, it's crucial to keep an eye on the sugar content in these beverages. Drinks high in added sugars, like regular soda, energy drinks, and soft drinks, can contribute excess calories to your diet. It's advisable to consume these beverages in moderation or avoid them altogether. Opting for healthier alternatives can support better hydration and overall health.

Stay Hydrated, Stay Healthy

To maintain proper hydration, one must be aware of specific indicators. You should be mindful if you rarely experience thirst and your urine is consistently colourless or light yellow. It's highly recommended to seek advice from a healthcare professional or a registered dietitian to establish the specific daily water intake that suits your needs. To uphold adequate hydration and prevent dehydration, it is advisable to prioritise water consumption as your primary beverage choice. Additionally, strive to incorporate the habit of drinking a glass of water with every meal, between meals, before, during, and after physical activity, and whenever you sense the need for hydration.

Risks of Overhydration

Generally, overconsumption of water is not a concern for healthy, well-nourished adults. However, athletes may be at risk of excessive water intake when preventing dehydration during prolonged or intense physical activity. When you drink excessive water, your kidneys may struggle to excrete the surplus, diluting the sodium levels in your blood. This condition, known as hyponatremia, can potentially become life-threatening and requires prompt medical attention. The human body's kidneys can process a maximum of 1 litre of water per hour. This means they can effectively remove only 0.8 to 1.0 litres of water per hour. It is important to note that excessive water intake can disrupt the body's electrolyte balance. While it is rare to accidentally consume too much water, it can occur, particularly during rigorous physical activities such as sports competitions or intense training sessions.

Hydration Tips for Professionals

Individual water intake needs can vary, and it is acceptable to adjust the intake based on personal preferences and lifestyle. For professionals with demanding work schedules or busy lifestyles, aiming for eight glasses of water daily can be a straightforward guideline to ensure adequate hydration. It is essential to understand that the ideal water intake varies for each individual based on their specific needs and circumstances. For additional guidance, seeking advice from a medical professional is advisable.

Hydration and Holistic Health

Human survival relies on the essential consumption of food and water, which are critical in maintaining overall well-being. Embracing a Prakriti-based diet is vital to achieving holistic health. Food provides the energy necessary for the body to function optimally, while adequate hydration from water is essential for supporting the various systems within the body. A well-rounded diet containing multiple nutrients and sufficient daily water intake is crucial for the proper functioning of the body's numerous physiological processes.

SUMMARY

Food: The Foundation of Life and Culture

Food is essential for survival, providing the energy and nutrients necessary for physical and cognitive development. It serves as a complex mix of chemical compounds, each playing a unique role in maintaining bodily functions and promoting overall health.

Beyond sustenance, food is a vital cultural connector. Culinary practices and rituals are integral to our identities and community bonds, reflecting the rich tapestry of human history.

Historically, the structure of meals has evolved, influenced by agriculture, societal norms, and industrialisation. The three-meal pattern—breakfast, lunch, and dinner—became standard as societies shifted from foraging to settled agriculture. Meals began to align with daily tasks, with communal dining being common. Over centuries, the timing and nature of meals varied, with breakfast emerging as a distinct meal in medieval Europe, often embraced by the upper classes.

In modern times, the formalisation of meal structures, particularly in the Victorian era, reinforced social status through etiquette and scheduling. Today, while breakfast, lunch, and dinner are widely observed, the timing and specifics vary based on cultural traditions and personal preferences. Moreover, dietary practices, such as those in Jainism, exemplify how spiritual beliefs influence meal timing and food choices. For instance, Jains consume their last meal before sunset to adhere to the principle of ahimsa, minimising harm to living beings.

Prakriti: Ayurveda and Nutritional Balance

In Ayurveda, food is categorised as an Earth Element, emphasising the importance of aligning dietary choices with one's Prakriti, or constitution. This concept recognises the intricate relationship between bodily structure and function, positing that optimised digestion leads to improved health. Ayurveda identifies three functional environments: Vata, Pitta, and Kapha, each influencing dietary needs.

Vata individuals require warm, moist foods to counterbalance dryness and coldness. Recommended foods include root vegetables, grains, and healthy oils. **Pitta** individuals thrive on cooling foods, such as leafy greens and moderate warmth, while avoiding excessively spicy dishes that may exacerbate their fiery nature. **Kapha** individuals benefit from light, dry foods to stimulate digestion and maintain balance, steering clear of heavy and cold items.

Understanding one's Prakriti is essential for optimal health, as it guides the selection of easily digestible foods tailored to individual needs. This holistic approach ensures a balanced lifestyle, emphasising progress in physical, mental, emotional, and spiritual health rather than perfection.

Water: Essential for Life

Hydration is crucial for overall well-being, with recommendations suggesting an average daily fluid intake of about 3.7 litres for men and 2.7 litres for women. However, individual requirements can vary based on factors like physical activity, climate, and health conditions. To prevent sleep disruptions, it's wise to avoid water consumption two hours before bedtime.

Adequate hydration enhances physical performance, sustains mental energy, and supports overall health. Water isn't the sole source of fluids; fruits, vegetables, and other beverages also contribute to hydration. Signs of proper hydration include infrequent thirst and light-coloured urine. Regularly drinking water with meals and throughout the day is crucial for maintaining optimal hydration levels.

In conclusion, food, Prakriti, and water are interconnected components that play vital roles in human health and well-being. Understanding and embracing these elements can lead to a more balanced, harmonious life.

Wisdom from Sacred Texts on Food, Water, and Health

Bhagavad Gita – The Three Categories of Food

In the Bhagavad Gita, food is classified according to the three gunas (qualities of nature): Sattva, Rajas, and Tamas. The Gita encourages the consumption of **Sattvic food,** which supports physical well-being, mental clarity, and spiritual growth.

Sattvic Food: Pure and nourishing foods like fresh fruits, vegetables, grains, and milk that are simple, clean, and easy to digest, promoting vitality and longevity.

Rajasic Food: Foods that are overly spicy, salty, or stimulating, such as fried or heavily seasoned dishes, leading to restlessness, agitation, and imbalance.

Tamasic Food: Stale, processed, or reheated foods that contribute to lethargy, confusion, and dullness in both body and mind.

(Source: Bhagavad Gita)

Ayurveda – Prakriti-Based Diet for Optimal Health

According to Ayurveda, food should align with an individual's **Prakriti** (constitution) to maintain balance and promote overall well-being. Ayurveda recognises three Prakriti types—Vata, Pitta, and Kapha—each with specific dietary guidelines:

Vata: People with a Vata constitution benefit from warm, moist, and nourishing foods that counterbalance dryness and cold.

Pitta: Cooling foods like fresh fruits, vegetables, and grains help soothe the heat in Pitta individuals.

Kapha: Light, dry, and warm foods are recommended to counteract heaviness and sluggishness in Kapha types. Balancing food intake based on one's Prakriti leads to mental, physical, and emotional harmony, aligning with the natural functioning of the body.

(Source: Ayurvedic Teachings)

Teachings of Prophet Muhammad – Drinking Water Slowly While Sitting

According to the teachings of Prophet Muhammad, drinking water slowly and while sitting has significant health benefits. The Prophet advised taking small sips rather than gulping water down in one go, with the following benefits:

Prevention of Choking: Drinking in a seated position helps water move down the throat correctly, preventing it from entering the windpipe and causing choking.

Improved Hydration: Slow sips while sitting allow the body to absorb water, enhancing hydration and facilitating smoother digestion.

Better Digestion: Drinking water too quickly can flood the stomach and dilute essential gastric juices. By sitting and drinking in moderation, digestion remains optimal, and issues like bloating are reduced.

This practice, supported by the Hadith, emphasises mindfulness and moderation in daily habits, fostering better health and well-being.

(Source: Hadith)

The Bible – The Necessity of Food and Water for Life

In Isaiah 49:10, the Bible underscores the essential role of food and water in human life:

"They shall not hunger nor thirst; neither shall the heat nor sun smite them: for he that hath mercy on them shall lead them, even by the springs of water shall he guide them."

This verse emphasises the importance of food, water, and shelter as fundamental for survival and well-being.

(Source: The Bible)

Buddhist Teachings – Water as a Symbol of Purity and the Role of Food in Community

In Buddhism, water symbolises purity and life, reflecting clarity and tranquillity. The practice of sharing food fosters community bonds, particularly through the tradition of almsgiving. During their daily rounds, monks receive food donations from laypeople, which highlights the interdependence between the community and the spiritual devotion of both the givers and receivers.

This practice emphasises the importance of generosity and mindfulness in sustaining not just the physical body but also the spiritual community as a whole.

(Source: Buddhist Teachings)

03

The Power of Mornings: Habits, Prayer & Reflection

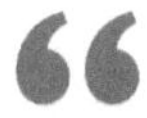

"In the morning, a man walks with his whole body; in the evening, only with his legs."

- Ralph Waldo Emerson.

Morning Magic: Habits for a Vibrant Start

Every person has a unique body type, and our bodies respond differently to waking up early. Some find it easy and comfortable, while others may feel tired, need more sleep, or struggle with laziness. Different individuals may rely on alarms or snooze buttons to wake up, while some program their minds before sleeping, enabling them to rise effortlessly. Techniques such as positive affirmations or subconscious messages can help foster a sense of purpose upon waking.

Within a family, each member often has their own routine. For instance, a husband's wake-up time may differ from a wife's, and children might follow their own schedules. Waking up in the morning with a refreshed body and mind is indeed a blessing. Ideally, the time spent sleeping should be free from the distractions of the digital world, allowing us to begin our day with spiritual practices right from our beds.

The Power of Gratitude

Before even opening your eyes, take a moment to express gratitude. Acknowledge the gift of a new day, your wonderful life, and the support of amazing parents, family, and friends. You might rub your palms together and bring them to your eyes before slowly opening them. Alternatively, simply take a brief moment to thank God for your caring parents, supportive family, close friends, and the comforts you have, including waking up on time. This practice of expressing gratitude only takes a few seconds but can significantly set a positive tone for your day. As William Arthur Ward wisely noted, "Gratitude can transform common days into thanksgivings, turn routine jobs into joy, and change ordinary opportunities into blessings." This simple act helps you start your day inspired and uplifted.

Breathing Techniques for Clarity

After expressing gratitude, practice an effective breathing technique. Begin by sitting comfortably on the edge of your bed and focusing on your breath. Place both hands near and just above your nose, then take a slow, deep breath, allowing your lungs to fill completely. Slowly exhale through your nose. Repeat this three times or as often as you feel comfortable, concentrating on how the breath enters and exits your body. You may notice that the air passes more easily through one nostril than the other, which is normal. This variation is an essential aspect of an ancient yogic practice known as **Swaravigyan**. It explores the flow of breath (swara) and its connection to the body's energy channels, or **nadis**. Understanding the breath's flow through the left nostril (Ida Nadi) and the right nostril (Pingala Nadi) allows you to align your energy with your body's natural rhythms.

Understanding Surya and Chandra Nadis

1. Surya Nadi (Pingala Nadi):

- **Associated with**: The right nostril.

- **Represents**: Solar energy (Surya means Sun), activity, heat, and masculine qualities.

- **Qualities**: Governs active energy, linked with logic and physical activity. It provides strength, energy, and warmth, encouraging action and outward movement.

- **When Active**: You may feel energetic and ready for tasks requiring focus and effort.

- **Effect on the Body**: Stimulates the sympathetic nervous system, increasing heart rate and body temperature.

2. Chandra Nadi (Ida Nadi):

- **Associated with**: The left nostril.

- **Represents**: Lunar energy (Chandra means Moon), calmness, coolness, and feminine qualities.

- **Qualities**: Connected with rest, creativity, and intuition, bringing peace and mental clarity.

- **When Active**: You may feel relaxed, calm, and focused on inner thoughts.

- **Effect on the Body**: Stimulates the parasympathetic nervous system, helping to slow the heart rate and promote relaxation.

Balancing Surya and Chandra Nadis

Practices like **Nadi Shodhana**, or alternate nostril breathing, help balance energy flow between Surya (Pingala) and Chandra (Ida) nadis. Achieving balance is vital for maintaining harmony between active and restful states in the body. When both nadis are balanced, energy flows through the **Sushumna Nadi**, leading to spiritual awakening and higher consciousness.

How to Practice Nadi Shodhana (Alternate Nostril Breathing)

1. **Find a Comfortable Position**: Sit comfortably in a cross-legged position (like Sukhasana) or on a chair, keeping your back straight and shoulders relaxed. Close your eyes to enhance focus.

2. **Set Your Hand Position (Vishnu Mudra)**: Use your right hand. Fold your index and middle fingers into your palm to form the Vishnu Mudra. Your thumb will block the right nostril, while your ring and little fingers will block the left nostril.

3. **Inhale through the Left Nostril**: Close the right nostril with your thumb and inhale slowly through the left nostril.

4. **Close the Left Nostril**: After inhaling completely through the left nostril, close it with your ring and little fingers so both nostrils are now closed.

5. **Exhale through the Right Nostril**: Release your thumb from the right nostril and exhale gently through the right side.

6. **Inhale through the Right Nostril**: Close the left nostril with your fingers and inhale deeply through the right nostril.

7. **Exhale through the Left Nostril**: Close the right nostril with your thumb. Open the left nostril and exhale completely through the left side.

This completes one round of Nadi Shodhana. Continue practicing this cycle for 5–10 minutes.

Enhancing Your Morning Practice

As you become more comfortable, gradually increase the duration or intensity of your practice. Nadi Shodhana is an excellent technique for calming the mind, balancing energy levels, and promoting clear breathing. It reduces stress and improves concentration, helping you start your day on a calm and balanced note. Remember, it's normal for it to take a few tries to master this technique. The key is to keep practising and discover what works best for you.

The Role of Restful Sleep in Energising Your Morning Routine

Waking up early often encourages an earlier bedtime, paving the way for a restorative night's sleep. Quality sleep offers numerous health benefits, including improved mental health, enhanced cognitive function, a stronger immune system, and a decreased risk of chronic health conditions. Research indicates that adequate sleep is essential for overall well-being, affecting mood, concentration, and physical health. It's important to note that the quality of sleep often matters more than the quantity; even a shorter duration of restful sleep can be more beneficial than a longer period of restless sleep. Our body's biological clock regulates various functions, including digestion and energy production, and aligns these processes with the natural light-dark cycle. Disrupting this rhythm by staying up late and waking up later can lead to misalignment, reducing the body's efficiency. Sleep is not just a time for rest; it activates essential restorative processes that repair muscles, tissues, and organs and clear waste products from the brain.

Morning Energy: Harnessing the Early Hours

The early morning hours, particularly from 4 AM to 7 AM, are often regarded as a time of heightened energy and productivity. During this period, the body is more receptive to various practices, including meditation, pranayama, physical exercise, and self-reflection, which can enhance mental clarity and emotional stability.

By engaging in these practices in the morning, you can capitalise on this unique energy, promoting inner balance and overall well-being. Missing this time of focused energy can mean forgoing opportunities for personal growth and productivity. By prioritising quality sleep and embracing early rising, you set the stage for a healthier, more fulfilling day.

Breaking the Habit of Time-Checking

It is common for many people to keep their mobile phones within close reach, and they constantly check notifications. Some individuals even develop the habit of frequently checking the time, which can adversely affect their well-being. Repeatedly looking at the watch can lead to increased anxiety and stress, disrupting focus and productivity at work or creating restlessness during sleep. When working, constantly checking the time breaks concentration, making tasks feel longer and more burdensome. During sleep, checking the time frequently can increase frustration and anxiety about not getting enough rest, making it harder to fall asleep again. This pattern can lead to a negative feedback loop, where the worry about time affects performance and relaxation. Avoiding frequent time checks helps maintain a calmer mindset and better time management. While getting enough sleep is crucial, constantly monitoring and worrying about the hours available for rest is not a healthy practice. Quality sleep is more important than quantity, and keeping digital devices at least 15-20 feet away from the bed or even out of the bedroom is recommended. Engaging in a complete digital detox an hour before sleep and an hour after waking up can significantly benefit one's overall well-being. Minimising exposure to blue light from screens improves sleep quality, reduces eye strain, prevents headaches, and helps maintain a healthy circadian rhythm, which supports better mental and physical well-being. Two hours of saved time from engaging in a digital detox can be utilised to participate in activities that boost productivity, as this time could be dedicated to activities such as exercise, reading, spending quality time with loved ones, yoga, meditation, or pursuing hobbies and interests. Embracing this opportunity can lead to a more balanced and fulfilling lifestyle.

The Importance of Making Your Bed

Starting your day by making your bed might appear a minor task, but it holds great significance in shaping your overall well-being. When you take the time to arrange your pillows, smooth out your sheets, and neatly prepare your bed, you are establishing a sense of order in your surroundings. This act, though simple, provides an immediate feeling of accomplishment. You have already achieved something right at the start of your day, which helps set a positive and productive tone. It creates the foundation for how the rest of your day will unfold. This small action can also act as a momentum builder. Completing this task early in the morning triggers a mental shift where you feel more prepared to handle other responsibilities. Taking care of one task, even as simple as making your bed, encourages you to tackle the rest of your day confidently and focus. It can spark a chain reaction where one task leads to another, allowing you to stay organised and manage your time effectively. Starting with this manageable step creates a sense of flow, making it easier to accomplish bigger tasks throughout the day.

Aside from productivity, making your bed can also positively impact your stress levels. After a long and busy day, coming home to a tidy, well-organised bed offers comfort and calm. The simple sight of a neat bed creates a relaxing atmosphere, helping you feel more at ease and providing a peaceful space to unwind. Keeping your environment organised can influence other areas of your home, encouraging you to maintain cleanliness and order throughout your living space, contributing to an overall sense of tranquillity. Over time, this daily habit of making your bed builds discipline and a sense of responsibility. While it may seem like a small routine, it reinforces the value of attention to detail and consistency. By practising this habit every day, you develop a mindset that values taking care of the small things in life. Often, it's those small actions that lead to bigger successes. The effort you put into maintaining this routine can spill over into other aspects of your life, helping you stay focused on larger goals and responsibilities. In essence, making your bed in the morning symbolises control over your environment and starts your day with a positive mindset. It is a practice that shows how small habits, when done regularly, can create a ripple effect of productivity, calmness, and self-discipline. By attending to this simple task, you appreciate how consistency and attention to small details can contribute to greater fulfilment and success throughout your life.

Morning Hydration: A Foundation for Well-Being

As you wake up, it's essential to prioritise hydrating your body. Find a peaceful spot to sit with your spine straight, whether it's on a cushion, on the floor, on a comfortable sofa, or on a supportive chair, and take the time to drink three glasses of room-temperature water (it may not be necessary for everyone). If you're finding it challenging to drink three glasses of water, reducing it to two or even one glass is also perfectly fine, which is the minimum suggested. A glass tumbler with a capacity of 250 ml is recommended for each serving. Staying adequately hydrated is essential for overall health, so finding a manageable routine that works for you is vital. This simple act of self-care has numerous benefits, such as aiding in eliminating toxins from your body, which can contribute to overall health and well-being. Additionally, drinking water upon waking can help dilute stomach acid, support better digestion, boost the immune system, and promote overall well-being. Doing so can improve the flow of nutrients to the brain and enhance brain activity. Furthermore, this seated position can also improve digestion and reduce the likelihood of feeling bloated. Drinking water in smaller sips while seated is recommended, allowing for better absorption and avoiding feeling uncomfortable or bloated. Additionally, it's advisable to avoid drinking water while standing, as this may not provide the same benefits as drinking while seated and may lead to less efficient hydration.

Post-Exercise Routines & Hot vs. Cold Showers

The preferences for post-exercise routines can differ from person to person, as individuals may choose to participate in activities like exercising, walking, or engaging in light physical workouts. After their physical training, some individuals like to follow up with a cup of coffee or tea before showering. Additionally, they may integrate meditation into their routine before bathing. However, engaging in meditation and prayers after bathing is generally suggested, as it promotes the purification of both the mind and body. If someone prefers to take a bath in the morning, opting for a cold bath can help invigorate and energise the body. Conversely, if a person is taking a bath at night, a hot bath can be more beneficial as it may promote relaxation and better sleep. The effectiveness of a cold-water bath can vary significantly depending on an individual's body type and constitution. While it offers numerous benefits, such as improved circulation, increased alertness, and enhanced immunity, it may not be suitable for everyone. For individuals who have a naturally colder body type or are more sensitive to temperature changes, suddenly introducing cold water baths may lead to discomfort, a drop in body temperature, or even symptoms like fever or a cold. Therefore, starting gradually and acclimatising the body to lower temperatures over time is important. People who are not accustomed to cold water exposure should begin with shorter durations and assess their body's response before making it a regular practice. If there are signs of discomfort, it's best to switch back to a warmer bath or consult a wellness practitioner. The key is to listen to your body's signals and adjust based on individual tolerance and health conditions.

Cold showers have been associated with several health benefits, including reducing inflammation, enhancing circulation, and lowering stress levels. In contrast, hot showers can promote relaxation, soothe muscles, and improve sleep quality. Knowing when to use hot or cold showers is essential for maximising their effects on the body and mind. Incorporating cold showers into a morning routine may lead to benefits; within a month, individuals might experience increased alertness, improved energy levels, better skin health, and enhanced mental well-being. Personally, I have observed a significant boost in my morning alertness and overall mood from this practice, making it an integral part of my daily routine.

Mastering the Art of Rising Early: Simple Adjustments

Some individuals may struggle with waking up early, and adapting to a sudden change in routine can be challenging. However, there are some simple strategies that can help ease this transition. One approach is gradually adjusting your wake-up time by 15 minutes each week. For instance, if you typically wake up at 7:00 AM, you can start by setting your alarm for 6:45 AM for the first week. The following week, you can put it for 6:30 AM and continue to shift your wake-up time earlier by 15-minute increments each week. By consistently adjusting your wake-up time in this manner, you can eventually work your way up to waking up an hour earlier. This incremental approach allows your body to gradually adapt to the change, making it easier to form a new habit of rising early. Consider setting short-term goals to achieve your desired rising time and practise this routine consistently for at least three months to instil **the habit of rising early.**

The next challenge is to break free from relying on alarms and snooze sounds and instead train your body to align with your natural waking rhythm, ultimately establishing a consistent daily routine. Owning pets can have the advantage of naturally waking you up from sleep. Training your body and mind to wake up at a specific time without an alarm is feasible. To improve your morning alertness, you can work on aligning your natural body clock, or circadian rhythm, by following these practical steps:

- **Understand Your Body's Clock**

Your body operates on a 24-hour cycle, which governs when you feel awake or sleepy. This clock is influenced by light, especially sunlight, and is crucial in regulating sleep and energy levels.

- **Get Morning Sunlight**

Stepping outside or opening your windows to natural light shortly after waking up signals to your brain that it's time to be alert. This helps adjust your internal clock, making mornings easier.

- **Stick to a Regular Sleep Routine**

Try to go to bed and wake up at the same time every day, even on weekends. This consistency trains your body to follow a natural rhythm, making it easier to wake up refreshed.

- **Exercise Regularly**

A morning workout, even a light one, can boost your energy levels for the entire day. Aim for at least 30 minutes of activity most days, which will also improve your sleep quality.

- **Create a Relaxing Evening Routine**

In the evening, dim your lights and avoid screens to let your body wind down naturally. Relaxing activities like reading or meditation can help you prepare for sleep. Avoid heavy meals or caffeine late in the day to prevent sleep disruption.

- **Tune Into Your Body's Signals**

Pay attention to when your body feels naturally tired. If you start feeling sleepy earlier in the evening, try going to bed instead of forcing yourself to stay up.

- **Be Patient with Changes**

Adjusting your body's internal clock won't happen overnight. Give yourself time to build these habits and stick to them consistently.

These steps will gradually train your body to feel more alert in the mornings and improve overall sleep quality.

Morning Harmony with Meditation and Movement

Meditation: Cultivating Calm and Clarity

Meditation can give you a sense of calm, peace, and balance that can benefit your emotional well-being and overall health. Focusing on something that calms you can help you relax and cope with stress. Meditation can also help you learn to stay centred and maintain inner peace. It involves a variety of practices aimed at sharpening attention, increasing emotional awareness, nurturing kindness, fostering compassion, promoting joy in the success of others, and cultivating mental serenity, even amid challenging or stressful situations. Regular meditation has been found to empower individuals to extend kindness to themselves and to show more care and empathy towards others. Going to a meditative state is difficult without regular practice, but simple steps done regularly can help you reach a meditative state over time. To start with, sit or lie comfortably. Sit in the meditation posture or lie on the bed, breathe deeply and evenly, and do not move. This means do not get up, fidget, change position, fix your hair, fix your outfit, or anything similar. Close your eyes and try not to control your breathing; breathe naturally. Focus on the breath and how the body moves with each inhalation and exhalation. With your eyes closed, breathe in while saying "breathe in" in your head as you do. Then breathe out and say, "Breathe out." Doing this for 3 to 5 minutes a week and gradually increasing it to 10 minutes for the next 20 minutes allows you to focus on this circular breath and the simple words in your head as much as possible. If necessary, you may listen to some soothing music, but ensure it is not too quiet, as you may strain to hear it. Listen to the music and let your thoughts fade away. Focus on the music: you should think of nothing but the music while meditating. If your thoughts stray, focus back on the music and stay there. Some people find listening to calming music for sleep or calming music for relaxation helps them focus and relax during meditation. However, others prefer complete silence to concentrate on their breath and thoughts better. Ideally, the morning is the best time for meditation. However, there are some other factors to consider, too. Meditation is often seen as a way of fixing the mind when it gets hectic or calming the body when stressed.

The Power of Daily Prayer: Nurturing Spiritual Connection

Born into a Hindu family, my spiritual journey has always been grounded in the customs and beliefs of Hinduism while maintaining deep respect for all religions and their practices. The focus of this journey is my faith in a higher power, which I call the Almighty God. Daily prayer and mantra recitation form an integral part of my routine.

The quiet of early morning offers an ideal time for prayers. It is a time when a unique energy can be felt, uplifting the spirit and bringing clarity. The calmness of the early hours promotes mental focus and inner peace, creating a sense of grounding for the day ahead. This serene time allows one to align thoughts and emotions, providing a refreshing and soothing start, which prepares the mind to face the challenges of the day with resilience and positivity.

Brahma Muhurta: The Creator's Time for Reflection

This time is known as Brahma Muhurta, which means "The Creator's Time." Brahma represents ultimate knowledge, and Muhurta refers to a specific time period. Brahma Muhurta is the best time to gain deep understanding and wisdom. It occurs between 3:30 AM and 5:30 AM or from around 3:40 AM until just before sunrise. During this period, the environment is calm and free from distractions, which enhances the quality of prayer and meditation. As the day progresses, our minds become filled with information, news, and conversations, making it hard to focus. However, when we wake up refreshed after a good night's sleep, our minds are more peaceful and less scattered. The air in the early morning is also fresh, with a higher oxygen content, which is scientifically beneficial for activities like yoga and breathing exercises. This clean air helps to improve our overall experience during these practices.

Harnessing Solar Energy: The Power of Sun Gazing and Surya Namaskara

In our pursuit of well-being, practices such as sun gazing and

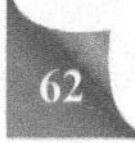

Surya Namaskara hold immense significance, both spiritually and physically. Sun gazing is a mindful practice that involves looking directly at the rising or setting sun, helping improve focus and achieve mental clarity. Advocates of this practice believe that the sun provides not only warmth and light but also energy and healing properties. Engaging in sun gazing with the right mindset fosters a deep connection with the divine light of the sun, creating a sense of spiritual harmony.

The Benefits of Sunlight and Vitamin D

Sunlight is essential for our bodies to produce vitamin D, often called the "sunshine vitamin." When our skin absorbs sunlight, it synthesises vitamin D from cholesterol, which is vital for maintaining healthy bones and muscles. Vitamin D also plays a significant role in regulating blood pressure, boosting the immune system, and reducing the risk of type 2 diabetes and certain cancers. Additionally, proper sunlight exposure can improve skin health and enhance overall vitality. Practising sun-gazing in the first 30-45 minutes after sunrise or before sunset, when the UV radiation is low, ensures the process remains safe for the eyes.

Surya Namaskara: A Complete Physical and Mental Workout

Surya Namaskara, or Sun Salutation, is a powerful sequence of yoga postures that have been practised for centuries to harness the benefits of the sun. Performing Surya Namaskara from 6 AM to 10 AM on an empty stomach is particularly effective, as it aligns the body and mind with nature's rhythm. This practice strengthens muscles and joints, enhances flexibility, improves circulation, and boosts immunity. It also aids in detoxification, supports weight loss, and contributes to glowing skin and healthy hair. Moreover, Surya Namaskara balances the mind and energises the body, making it a holistic practice for overall wellness.

Sun gazing and Surya Namaskara offer a harmonious blend of spiritual and physical benefits. By integrating these practices into your daily routine, you can harness the energy of the sun to nurture both body and mind, fostering a healthier, more balanced life.

Maintaining Routine: Balancing Work and Leisure

Many people tend to embrace a more laid-back and unhurried lifestyle on weekends and holidays compared to their regular weekday schedule. This often involves sleeping in, enjoying a leisurely brunch instead of the usual hurried breakfast, and following a more adaptable and relaxed daily routine. Whether this change in routine is beneficial or detrimental is a frequently debated topic, and the answer can be found here. It is important to stick to your daily routine, even on weekends. Your daily routine is crucial in helping you stay organised and accomplish your tasks. By managing all your weekend chores in one day, you can free up the rest of the weekend to relax and recharge. Completing your daily chores all at once gives you more leisure time to enjoy activities such as watching movies, unwinding, working out, and spending time with friends. This approach will rejuvenate you and make your weekend much more fulfilling. Instead of spending an entire day on cleaning and laundry, consider consolidating these tasks to make more time for yourself.

Consistency and Variation: Keys to a Fulfilling Life

Many successful individuals adhere to strict daily routines in their regular practice. A daily routine is beneficial as it helps regulate energy levels, thus minimising daily fluctuations. This consistency positively impacts productivity and acts as a buffer against stress. The disciplined approach allows for better time management, creating the opportunity to focus more on work and fostering an environment that encourages regular idea generation. Adhering to a consistent routine during the weekdays can be beneficial, but it's essential to introduce some variation during the weekends. Many embark on a week-long getaway to engage in activities they've never experienced. This serves as an effective strategy for preventing life from becoming monotonous. While on vacation, it's essential to allocate some time for relaxation and personal reflection. This facilitates mental and emotional rejuvenation, leaving you more invigorated upon your return. Additionally, spending time with family and friends and participating in preferred activities are integral to a fulfilling weekend. Ultimately, the objective is to ensure that your weekends differ from your weekday routine. Varying your schedule is critical for staving off boredom and promoting the overall health of your body and mind.

Strategies for Staying Motivated: Building Momentum

Having a focused goal and a straightforward routine is very important. When you set a goal—whether it is earning a degree, getting a new job, or improving your physical fitness—you are making a big move towards improving your life. However, staying committed and following through can be tough, especially when your motivation decreases over time. Feeling enthusiastic when setting a goal is natural, but that excitement can fade as challenges arise or progress seems slow. This is where discipline and routine come into play. Sticking to a consistent plan, even on days when you don't feel like it, makes all the difference. A routine helps you maintain focus, keeps you on track, and ensures that you make steady progress.

In India, we often see the power of dedication in different walks of life. Whether it is a student preparing for competitive exams or a sportsperson training to win a medal, the journey involves hard work and persistence. Just like them, if you keep moving forward one step at a time, even small efforts add up over time and help you reach your goal.

Here are some science-backed strategies that can help you stay on track, even when you're feeling unmotivated:

- **Schedule Your Goal:** Marking your goal on a calendar makes it feel more real and helps you stay accountable. It turns your plan into something tangible and encourages you to follow through.

- **Build a Habit:** Incorporate actions towards your goal into your daily routine. Working towards it regularly becomes a natural part of your day and requires less effort over time.

- **Prepare for Setbacks:** Challenges are inevitable in any journey. Having a plan to handle obstacles ensures that you can bounce back more easily when setbacks occur.

- **Set Small Milestones:** Breaking your bigger goal into smaller, manageable steps makes it less overwhelming. Achieving these milestones provides momentum and keeps your motivation high.

- **Monitor Your Progress:** Keeping track of your achievements through journaling or an app helps you stay focused. Regular progress updates allow you to see how far you've come.

- **Celebrate Successes:** Rewarding yourself for each milestone, no matter how small, boosts your motivation. These rewards encourage us to continue pushing forward.

- **Surround Yourself with Positivity:** The people around you play a huge role in your success. Stay connected with those who inspire and encourage you, helping you stay committed to your goals.

- **Daily Agenda Setting:** Creating a to-do list or outlining tasks for the day helps prioritise important activities, ensuring nothing is overlooked. It provides structure to the day, enabling better time management. This approach boosts productivity by maintaining focus and reducing procrastination.

- **Practice Gratitude:** Reflect on your efforts and appreciate your progress. Being thankful for the journey itself cultivates positivity and keeps you motivated.

- **Uplift Your Mood:** Engage in activities that energise and refresh you. A positive mindset helps you stay motivated and focused on achieving your goal.

- **Change Your Environment:** A new environment can provide fresh motivation. Changing your surroundings can sometimes re-energise you and help you refocus on your goal.

- **Reflect on Your Purpose:** Remind yourself why you set the goal in the first place. Reconnecting with your reasons reignites your passion and commitment, pushing you closer to success. Reflect on your **"why."**

These strategies can help you navigate times of low motivation, keep you on track toward achieving your goals, and maintain a consistent daily routine. **The habit of rising early** can lead to overall well-being. With these practices, an aligned body, mind, and emotions will keep us healthy, wealthy, and wise!

SUMMARY

Morning Habits Overview:

Individual Differences in Waking Up:

- People have varying body types and responses to waking up early; some feel energised, while others may need more sleep.

- Some rely on alarms, while others use mental programming or positive affirmations to wake up purposefully.

Family Routines:

- Each family member may have a different waking schedule, highlighting the importance of understanding personal routines.

Morning Gratitude:

- Starting the day with gratitude can set a positive tone. Simple practices like thanking God for a new day can transform one's mindset.

Breathing Techniques:

- Engaging in breathing exercises upon waking, such as Swaravigyan, aligns the body's energy with natural rhythms and enhances mental clarity.

Nadi Shodhana (Alternate Nostril Breathing):

- This technique balances the energy channels (Surya Nadi and Chandra Nadi) in the body, promoting overall well-being.

Benefits of Early Wakefulness:

- Waking up early can enhance sleep quality, mental health, and immune function, aligning the body's natural clock with energy cycles.

Digital Detox:

- Minimising screen time for 1 hour before bedtime and after waking can improve sleep quality and reduce anxiety.

Making the Bed:

- This small task instils a sense of accomplishment and order, positively influencing productivity and stress levels throughout the day.

Hydration:

- Drinking water in the morning aids digestion, flushes toxins, and supports overall health.

Post-Exercise Routines:

- Individuals may have various preferences, including meditation and post-exercise, with recommendations for optimal timing.

Cold Showers:

- These can boost alertness and mood, with individual tolerance crucial for acclimatisation.

Adjusting Wake-Up Times:

- Gradually shifting wake-up times can help individuals adapt to earlier rising, promoting better habits and natural rhythms.

Meditation and Prayer:

- Meditation fosters calmness, balance, and emotional well-being. It helps individuals stay centred and cultivate kindness and compassion.

- Regular practice can enhance focus and mental serenity. Beginners can start by sitting comfortably, breathing deeply, and concentrating on their breath, gradually increasing the duration of practice.

- Morning meditation and prayer during **Brahma Muhurta** (3:30 AM to 5:30 AM) is ideal, as the environment is peaceful and conducive to spiritual practices.

Sun Gazing and Physical Practices:

- Sun gazing, performed safely at sunrise or sunset, is believed to improve focus and energy while promoting vitamin D production, which benefits overall health.

- **Suryanamaskara**, practised on an empty stomach, strengthens muscles, boosts immunity, and promotes overall well-being.

Daily Routine and Goal Setting:

- Maintaining a consistent daily routine, even on weekends, enhances productivity and time management, allowing for more leisure time.

- It's essential to introduce variation during weekends to prevent monotony and promote overall mental and emotional health.

- Setting clear goals and adhering to a routine helps maintain focus and discipline, even when motivation wanes.

- Create a to-do list or outline tasks to prioritise daily activities and avoid overlooking essential tasks. It provides structure, boosts productivity, and improves time management.

Strategies for Motivation:

- Effective strategies include scheduling goals, building habits, preparing for setbacks, setting small milestones, tracking progress, celebrating successes, surrounding oneself with positivity, practising gratitude, uplifting mood, changing environments, and reflecting on one's purpose.

Incorporating these practices can lead to a healthier, more fulfilling life, aligning the body, mind, and emotions.

04

Rituals for Daily Magic

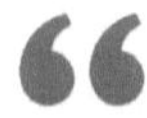

A daily routine built on good habits and disciplines separates the most successful among us from everyone else.

- Darren Hardy

As mentioned in the previous chapters, having a digital detox one hour before bed and one hour after waking up is essential. A simple diet that is good for our body and mind continuously improves overall well-being. Once you establish **the habit of rising early**, you set yourself up for a successful day. To optimise your mornings and extend the benefits throughout the day, you should integrate the following rituals into your daily routine.:

1. Affirmation

2. Gratitude

3. Imagination

4. Visualisation

5. Vision Board

6. Exercise

7. Reading & The Value of Writing

8. Intermittent Fasting

9. Creating a Balanced and Fulfilling Lifestyle Through Gardening and Tree Planting

10. The Importance of Silence

11. Integrating Acts of Kindness, Forgiveness and Acceptance

12. The Transformative Power of Music

In the pursuit of overall well-being, it's important to prioritise various activities that contribute to a healthy mind and body. This includes incorporating affirmations, expressing gratitude, engaging in imaginative thinking and visualisation, and dedicating time to reading into our daily routines. Additionally, we shouldn't overlook the benefits of gardening, as it offers physical activity and stimulates the mind. Just as physical exercise is essential for our bodies, these cognitive activities are indispensable for nurturing and maintaining a sharp and active mind.

AFFIRMATION

An affirmation is a powerful psychological technique that involves repeating positive statements to reprogram the subconscious mind. These statements serve to challenge and replace negative or self-limiting beliefs, promoting a more optimistic and confident mindset. By reinforcing positive thinking patterns, affirmations can profoundly impact one's overall well-being and success.

Key Features of Affirmations

- Stay Positive: Always positively write affirmations. Focus on what you want to achieve or believe instead of what you want to avoid. This can help change negative thoughts and encourage a positive attitude.

- **Present Focus:** Use the present tense for your affirmations, as if what you desire is already happening.

This helps your mind accept the belief more easily. By thinking about the present, affirmations feel more real and encourage your subconscious to believe them.

- **Daily Practice:** For effective affirmations, repeat them daily. Saying positive statements regularly can help replace negative or limiting beliefs with more encouraging ones. This habit can lead to a long-lasting change in your mindset over time.

- **Build Self-Empowerment:** Affirmations allow you to focus on your strengths, goals, and positive traits. They can improve your self-esteem, reduce doubts, and help you stay positive. By focusing on self-empowerment, affirmations can strengthen your belief in yourself and boost your confidence and well-being.

Benefits of Using Affirmations in Your Daily Life

- **Boosts Self-Confidence:** Regularly using positive statements can help reduce self-doubt and increase your self-esteem, making you feel more confident in yourself.

- **Reduced Stress and Anxiety:** By frequently telling yourself positive things, you can shift your negative thoughts and develop a more hopeful outlook. This can help lower your stress and anxiety levels.

- **Increased Motivation and Focus:** Adding affirmations to your daily routine can help you consistently remember your goals. This can provide strong motivation and help you stay focused on what you want to achieve.

- **Support for Emotional Healing:** Affirmations are valuable for emotional healing. They can help change negative beliefs and past experiences, leading to personal growth and resilience.

Affirmations are a powerful tool that can significantly impact your thoughts, actions, and overall well-being.

Simple Steps to Practice Affirmations Effectively

Step 1: Choose Your Affirmation

Start by selecting a positive affirmation that deeply resonates with your goals or aspirations. Ensure that the affirmation reflects how you want to feel or what you want to achieve. For it to have a meaningful impact, you must feel empowered and connected to it.

Examples:

- "I am confident, capable, and worthy of success."

  "I embrace abundance and growth in all areas of my life."

- "I am healthy, energetic, and strong."

Step 2: Use the Present Tense

Your affirmation should be worded as if it's happening now. By using phrases like "I am" or "I have," you train your subconscious mind to view your desired outcomes as current realities. Keep the language positive and focused on what you want rather than what you don't want.

Step 3: Speak It Out Loud

Saying your affirmation out loud with conviction can amplify its effect. You may find it helpful to stand in front of a mirror, make eye contact with yourself, and repeat the affirmation 3-5 times in each session. Focus on genuinely feeling the words as you speak to them.

Step 4: Visualise the Desired Outcome

While reciting your affirmation, picture the outcome as if it's already happening. Visualise yourself achieving success and joy or calm your desire. Fully engage in this visualisation by allowing yourself to experience the emotions tied to the fulfilment of your affirmation.

Step 5: Make It a Daily Practice

Consistency is key to making affirmations effective. Incorporate them into your daily routine, especially during the morning, to set a positive tone for the day and before bed to anchor your mindset. Over time, repetition reinforces your belief in the affirmation, gradually leading to personal growth and positive change.

GRATITUDE

Gratitude is about embracing the feeling of thankfulness and expressing appreciation for the positive elements in our lives, regardless of their size. It involves acknowledging and valuing the support from others and finding joy and value in our experiences. Gratitude emphasises being aware of the blessings we have received and taking the time to savour and appreciate the present moment for what it is. Gratitude is a powerful emotion that can displace negative feelings such as fear, anxiety, shame, and worry, as well as more toxic emotions like ego and hate. When we cultivate gratitude, we pave the way for a profound sense of happiness and contentment. It's essential to recognise that while weeds may flourish effortlessly, cultivating a beautiful garden filled with roses requires dedicated effort. Similarly, fostering gratitude is necessary for nurturing the blessings in our lives.

Gratitude transcends mere thankfulness for the apparent aspects of life, such as having a place to live, access to food, clean water, and the presence of friends and family. It's about reflecting on our fortunes whenever something positive occurs, regardless of its magnitude. Gratitude encourages us to appreciate the richness of our lives rather than constantly seeking external sources of happiness or remaining fixated on unmet material and physical needs. By acknowledging and embracing gratitude, we can shift our focus from what is lacking to a more profound appreciation of our abundance.

Every morning, when you start your day by expressing gratitude for the simple things in life. Awakening to a new day and the ability to breathe are precious gifts we often take for granted. Taking the time to appreciate the air we breathe, the water we drink, the food we eat, and the sleep we receive each night can bring a sense of contentment and mindfulness to our lives. Additionally, acknowledging the significance of the sunlight we receive from the sun, which provides us with blessings and energy, helps us develop a deeper appreciation for the world around us. It's essential to be thankful for our body, mind, and all our senses, as well as the gift of good health. Furthermore, it's worth contemplating the importance of growth and contribution. Many successful individuals, including millionaires and business tycoons, continue to work without retirement because they recognise that growth and contribution are key elements of their prosperity. On the other hand, individuals facing financial hardship may focus primarily on monetary concerns. This dichotomy underscores the differing perspectives on life and success between the wealthy and the less fortunate.

Key Aspects of Gratitude

- **Appreciating the Present:** Gratitude helps you focus on the present moment, allowing you to find happiness in what you have right now instead of always wanting more. It encourages you to recognise and be thankful for the good things in your current situation, bringing you peace and satisfaction.

- **Recognising the Good in Life:** Gratitude means acknowledging and valuing the good things in life. This can come from others, like the kindness of friends, or from your own growth and achievements. By actively appreciating these positives, you create a more positive mindset and improve your overall well-being.

- **Building Positive Relationships:** Showing gratitude can strengthen your connections with others. By expressing appreciation for the support and kindness you receive, you enhance your relationships and create a caring, supportive environment.

- **Practicing Mindfulness:** Gratitude encourages you to be more aware of the often-overlooked aspects of life that contribute to your happiness. This includes recognising small things, like good health, the beauty of nature, or simple acts of kindness. By being more mindful and appreciative, you can find greater joy and fulfilment in your daily life.

Examples of Gratitude

- **Be Thankful for Loved Ones:** Appreciate your family, friends, and loved ones who support and stand by you.

- **Value Your Opportunities:** Recognise the chances you have, like education, a job, or the freedom to follow your passions.

- **Enjoy Small Moments:** Find joy in everyday experiences, like a beautiful sunset, a tasty meal, or a kind act from someone.

- **Learn from Challenges:** Feel thankful for personal challenges because they help you learn and grow.

Benefits of Practicing Gratitude

- **Better Mental Health:** Being grateful can improve mental health by reducing stress, anxiety, and depression. Focusing on what you appreciate helps shift your mindset to a more positive outlook on life.

- **More Happiness:** Regularly expressing gratitude is linked to higher levels of happiness and overall life satisfaction. It helps you understand what brings contentment and fulfilment.

- **Stronger Relationships:** Showing gratitude can enhance your relationships by promoting positive interactions and deeper connections. Appreciating others strengthens bonds and increases feelings of closeness.

- **Increased Resilience:** Gratitude can help you cope with tough situations. By focusing on the positives, even during hard times, you can build resilience and find strength to overcome challenges.

- **Better Physical Health:** Grateful people often experience better physical health. Research shows gratitude can lead to lower blood pressure, better sleep, a stronger immune system, and higher self-esteem, benefiting overall health.

Ways to Practice Gratitude

- **Morning Reflection:** Before getting out of bed, close your eyes and think about the day ahead. Be thankful for simple things like the new day, your health, your loved ones, and the comfort of your bed. This peaceful practice can help you start your day with a positive mindset.

- **Gratitude Journal:** Keep a journal where you write down things you're grateful for every day, no matter how small. This practice helps you focus on the positive aspects of your life, even during tough times.

- **Gratitude Meditation:** Spend a few moments each day meditating on things you appreciate in life. This could be a special person, a positive experience, or anything that brings you joy.

- **Express Thanks:** Take time to thank the people around you. Whether it's a simple "thank you" or a heartfelt letter, expressing gratitude can deepen your connections and bring joy to others.

- **Mindful Appreciation:** Be present and aware of your surroundings. Take time to enjoy moments of joy, beauty, or kindness as they happen. This practice can help you cultivate deeper gratitude for the world around you.

In essence, gratitude is a powerful practice that can transform your perspective, leading to a more fulfilled, joyful, and balanced life. It fosters positivity and contentment by recognising the abundance of goodness in everyday moments.

IMAGINATION

"Imagination is more important than knowledge.
For knowledge is limited to all we now know and understand,
while imagination embraces the entire world, and all there
ever will be to know and understand."

— Albert Einstein

Imagination is the ability of the mind to form images, ideas, sensations, or concepts that are not present to the senses. It allows you to think beyond the immediate and tangible reality, creating mental scenarios, exploring possibilities, and envisioning things that don't exist in the present moment. Imagination is crucial in creativity, problem-solving, innovation, and even empathy.

"Everything we see around us on planet Earth is the result of someone, somewhere, first imagining it and then setting out to make it a reality. Take a book, for example. It starts with someone imagining the story and its characters in their mind. Then, through the writing process, those thoughts are translated into words and pages, bringing the book to life. This is just one example of how most creations begin with imagination. If imagination is the secret to success, why don't more of us actively imagine the lives we desire to lead and the impact we want to make? Imagining the future we want to create can be the first step toward achieving it. Whether it's picturing the life we want to build or the lifestyle we want to embody, imagination plays a crucial role in shaping our reality. In essence, imagination involves envisioning things that are beyond our current reality to become the best version of ourselves. This could mean achieving financial abundance, positively impacting the lives of others, becoming a champion in our field, or simply striving to be the best version of ourselves. Imagination can be seen as a powerful tool that can transform our self-image and help us reach new heights."

Key Aspects of Imagination

- Visual Thinking: Imagination allows us to form detailed

mental images, letting us envision hypothetical situations, future events, and even entirely made-up worlds. This mental "vision" provides a way to explore new ideas and scenarios beyond the present reality.

- Innovative Ideation: Imagination is the foundation of innovation. It encourages us to break boundaries, invent creative solutions, and come up with fresh ideas. Whether in art, writing, music, or design, imagination drives the creative process that leads to groundbreaking work.

- Creative Problem-Solving: Imaginative thinking enables us to approach problems from different angles, explore alternative solutions, and foresee potential outcomes. It's a key tool for developing innovative answers to challenges that require out-of-the-box thinking.

- Emotional Insight: Imagination gives us the ability to understand and emotionally connect with others by visualising their feelings and experiences. This fosters empathy and helps deepen interpersonal relationships through shared understanding.

- Vision for the Future: Imagination is crucial in planning for the future and setting goals. By mentally projecting ourselves into future situations, we can picture what success looks like and use that vision as a powerful motivator toward achieving our objectives.

- Exploration of Fantasy: Daydreams and fantasies are another form of imagination, allowing us to mentally escape the confines of reality. Through this mental journey, we can explore desires, ideas, and scenarios beyond the real world, providing both inspiration and personal reflection.

Imagination Types: As shown in the below figure

1. Effectuative Imagination – Synthesising information together to form new concepts and ideas.

2. Intellectual (or Constructive) – A deliberate process of working from plans towards a distinct purpose.

3. Dreams – Unconscious images, ideas, emotions, and sensations that occur during certain stages of sleep

4. Emotional Imagination – Projecting emotional dispositions into external scenarios.

5. Strategic Imagination – The wisdom to understand the potential & limitations of possible scenarios

6. Empathy Imagination – Know emotionally what others are experiencing

7. Fantasy Imagination – Generating new ideas for art, literature, music, etc.

8. Memory Reconstruction – Retrieving our memory of people, objects, and events.

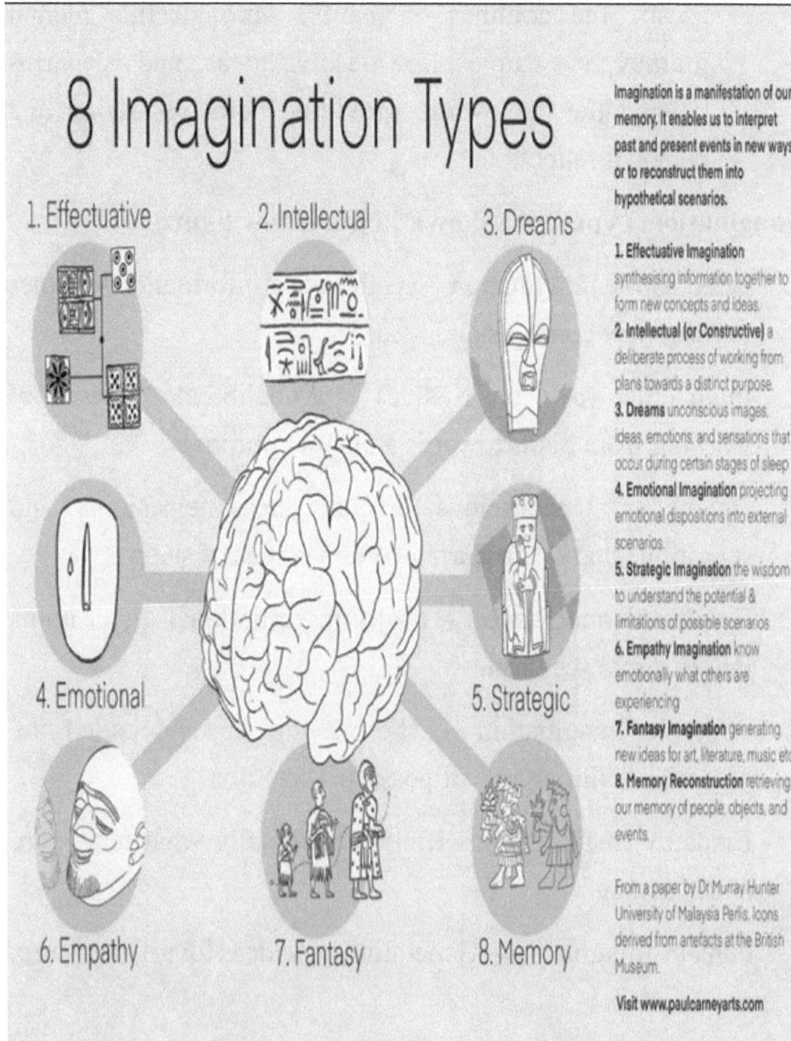

The Importance of Imagination

- Ignites Creativity: Imagination is the spark behind innovative business ideas, captivating stories, and unique product designs. It allows for the creation of something new and original.

- Fuels Innovation: By pushing the boundaries of what's possible, imagination plays a key role in driving scientific discoveries and technological advancements, leading to progress in countless fields.

- Strengthens Cognitive Abilities: Imagination is essential for developing mental faculties such as memory, critical thinking, and visualisation. It helps train the mind to think in diverse ways, boosting overall cognitive performance.

- Boosts Emotional Resilience: Imagination offers comfort and inspiration, helping individuals cope with challenges, envisioning hopeful futures, and enhancing their emotional well-being.

- Enhances Learning: By connecting abstract concepts to real-world situations, imagination facilitates deeper understanding and aids in grasping complex ideas, making learning more engaging and meaningful.

Examples of Imagination in Action

- Creating Art: Artists imagine a scene in their mind before painting.

- Telling Stories: Authors create characters, settings, and plots by imagining them.

- Being Innovative: Inventors imagine new tools or technology to solve problems or enhance lives.

- Showing Empathy: Imagining a friend's feelings after a tough experience helps you provide support and understanding.

- Visualising Goals: Envisioning yourself to achieve a goal can motivate and guide your actions.

VISUALISATION

Visualisation is a dynamic mental tool that involves forming vivid, detailed images or scenarios in the mind. By using the imagination to simulate experiences, individuals can mentally rehearse goals or outcomes as if they were happening in reality. This technique is widely applicable in areas such as achieving personal goals, enhancing performance, reducing stress, and preparing for future events. When individuals tap into the power of visualisation, they often find themselves more motivated, focused, and confident in pursuing their desired outcomes.

Key Aspects of Visualisation

- Cognitive Imagery: Visualisation involves the mental creation of vivid, detailed images or scenarios, whether they're based on real experiences or purely imagined situations. By engaging multiple senses and emotions, it creates a rich and immersive experience in the mind.

- Focused Goal Setting: Many people use visualisation as a tool to concentrate on specific goals, imagining themselves succeeding in personal or professional pursuits. Athletes, for instance, often visualise performing successfully before an event, helping them mentally prepare and simulate their optimal performance.

- Fostering a Positive Mindset: Visualisation is an effective way to build positive thinking and self-confidence. By rehearsing success mentally and envisioning positive outcomes, individuals can reduce anxiety, increase self-belief, and maintain a more empowered mental state.

- Sensory and Emotional Engagement: Effective visualisation goes beyond visual images; it involves immersing oneself fully by engaging all senses—imagining how things feel, sound, smell, and look. This adds depth to the mental practice, making it more impactful and realistic.

- Linking Mind and Body: Research has shown that mental rehearsal can activate neural pathways in the brain, much like physically performing the action. This mind-body connection is why athletes, performers, and even individuals working on personal growth use visualisation to sharpen their skills and improve their performance.

Practical Ways to Visualise

- Envision Success: Mentally imagine achieving personal or professional goals by visualising a successful outcome and mentally rehearsing the steps needed to get there.

- Performance Rehearsal: Athletes, musicians, and performers often practice their routines mentally before an event. This technique helps improve confidence and strengthens muscle memory by engaging the mind in the same way the body would during the actual performance.

- Healing Imagery: Visualisation can also be used in the healing process, where individuals imagine their body recovering from illness or injury. This practice is often integrated into holistic or alternative health approaches.

- Guided Visualisation: In many relaxation or goal-setting exercises, individuals follow a guided script, recording, or instructor-led session designed to lead them through specific visualisation scenarios, such as achieving goals or enhancing well-being.

- Stress Relief and Calming Scenes: Visualising peaceful, serene environments, such as beaches or forests, can provide a mental escape from stress, helping reduce anxiety and promoting a sense of calm.

Benefits of Visualisation

- **Increased Focus and Motivation:** Regularly visualising your goals strengthens your commitment to achieving them. This mental reinforcement enhances your ability to maintain focus and stay motivated, increasing the likelihood of success.

- **Enhanced Performance:** Visualisation is commonly used by athletes, performers, and professionals to mentally rehearse their skills. This type of mental practice improves physical performance and boosts confidence, leading to better outcomes.

- **Anxiety Reduction:** By visualising positive outcomes or calm environments, individuals can effectively reduce anxiety in stressful situations. Visualisation fosters a sense of control, creating a calming effect that lowers anxiety levels.

- **Improved Problem-Solving**: Visualisation enables individuals to mentally explore different strategies and solutions. By simulating possible outcomes, they can anticipate challenges and navigate them more effectively, leading to better problem-solving abilities.

- **Increased Confidence**: Visualising success and accomplishment helps build self-confidence. When individuals regularly picture themselves achieving their goals, they reinforce their belief in their abilities, leading to greater confidence.

Examples of Visualisation in Action

- Athletes: Prior to a basketball game, a player may visualise making free throws to enhance their muscle memory and concentration.

- Public Speaking: A speaker can picture themselves delivering a compelling presentation, imagining the audience's positive responses, and experiencing feelings of calm and confidence throughout their talk.

- Personal Goals: To maintain motivation and focus, an individual can visualise achieving a fitness milestone, such as finishing a marathon or reaching a particular weight target.

- Stress Relief: Envisioning a tranquil setting, like a peaceful beach or a quiet forest, can help soothe the mind and alleviate stress during anxious moments.

How to Practice Visualisation

- Get Comfortable: Find a quiet space, close your eyes, and take deep breaths to help relax your body.

- Picture Clearly: Focus on a specific goal, event, or experience that you wish to visualise. Strive to make the image as vivid and detailed as possible.

- Use Your Imagination: Engage all your senses by imagining what you see, hear, feel, smell, or taste. This enhances the realism of the visualisation.

- Imagine Success: Visualise yourself achieving your goal or excelling in the task at hand. Picture the steps you will take and the feelings of achievement and satisfaction that follow.

- Repeat Regularly: Practice visualisation consistently, whether daily or before particular events. Regularity increases the effectiveness of visualisation over time.

Visualisation is a powerful mental tool. It helps you picture outcomes, build confidence, and prepare for success. Visualisation can mentally prepare you for future events by bridging the gap between imagination and reality, whether you want to achieve goals, improve performance, or reduce stress.

VISION BOARD

A vision board is an effective tool designed to inspire and direct the mind by harnessing the powers of visualisation and imagination. It consists of a collection—either physical or digital—of images, words, and symbols that represent your goals, dreams, and aspirations. The primary purpose of a vision board is to act as a daily reminder of what you want to achieve, helping you maintain focus on those objectives.

1. Visualisation

Visualisation involves mentally picturing your desired outcomes or future aspirations. A vision board enhances this process by providing a visual focal point that you can regularly engage with. By observing the images, phrases, or symbols on your board, your mind becomes conditioned to perceive your goals as more concrete and achievable. This technique leverages the psychology of positive reinforcement, allowing you to feel a stronger connection to your goals each time you interact with the board.

For example, if your goal is to purchase a new home, you might include pictures of houses or home interiors on your board. Each time you see these images, you subconsciously strengthen your belief that achieving this goal is possible. The visualisation facilitated by a vision board boosts your motivation and readiness to take action, as it centres on your dreams and renders them more attainable.

2. Imagination

Imagination involves engaging the creative aspects of your mind. As you create your vision board, you give yourself the freedom to dream and reflect on what you genuinely desire in life. This exercise encourages you to think about the practical steps necessary to reach your goals and envision how to live a fulfilling, vibrant life.

While gathering images and words for your board, you utilise your imagination to construct a vision of your ideal future. It prompts you to ask questions like, "What does my perfect day look like?" or "What will I feel like when I achieve this goal?" This process activates the creative regions of your brain, aiding in the crystallisation of your desires and ambitions.

The Synergy of Visualization and Imagination

The true power of a vision board lies in its ability to combine visualisation and imagination into a focused experience. By regularly engaging with your vision board, you consistently stimulate your mind to visualise the life you aspire to while also encouraging imaginative thinking about other desires and possibilities that may arise.

When you interact with your vision board consistently, it can lead to several significant outcomes:

- **Clarifies Intentions**: It compels you to specify your goals and focus on what genuinely matters to you.

- **Fosters Motivation**: Daily reminders of your aspirations can propel you to take actionable steps toward your objectives.

- **Activates the Law of Attraction**: Many believe that concentrating on what you want helps draw those things into your life. While the scientific basis for this is debated, the mental alignment between your desires and actions is undeniable.

The Importance of Emotional Connection

A vision board also taps into the emotional dimension of visualisation. When you view images that resonate with your goals, they evoke emotions—such as excitement, hope, and passion—that align with the future you are working toward. These feelings energise you and propel you forward, making the board an active component of your journey toward personal growth and success rather than just a passive tool.

In summary, a vision board is more than merely a collection of pictures; it is a dynamic instrument that integrates visualisation and imagination to keep your mind aligned with your goals, encourage consistent effort, and inspire creativity in your pursuit of aspirations.

EXERCISE

Physical exercise encompasses any activity that is intentionally planned, organised, and executed with the primary aim of enhancing or maintaining physical fitness, health, and overall well-being. This includes a wide variety of movements designed to improve cardiovascular health, build muscle strength, increase flexibility, and promote mental wellness. From simple actions like walking and stretching to more vigorous activities such as weightlifting, running, or engaging in sports, exercise comes in many forms and intensities, catering to diverse preferences and fitness levels. Regular participation in physical exercise offers individuals numerous benefits associated with a healthy and active lifestyle.

Key Types of Exercise

- **Aerobic Exercise (Cardiovascular Exercise)**: This type of exercise involves activities that elevate your heart rate and increase your breathing for a sustained period. It helps strengthen the heart and lungs and improves blood circulation throughout the body. Common examples of aerobic exercise include running, swimming, cycling, brisk walking, and dancing.

- **Strength Training (Resistance Exercise)**: Strength training focuses on building and toning muscles through weights or other forms of resistance. It enhances muscle strength, endurance, and bone health. Examples of strength training exercises include weight lifting, push-ups, using resistance bands, and bodyweight exercises.

- **Flexibility and Stretching**: Flexibility and stretching exercises are essential for improving joint and muscle mobility, helping to prevent injuries. Some examples include yoga, Pilates, dynamic stretching, and static stretches.

- **Balance and Coordination Exercises**: These exercises enhance stability, improve movement efficiency, and increase body awareness. They are particularly important for older adults to reduce the risk of falls. Examples include Tai Chi, balance exercises, and standing on one leg.

- **High-Intensity Interval Training (HIIT)**: HIIT involves alternating between short bursts of intense exercise and brief periods of rest or lower-intensity activity. This training method is effective for improving cardiovascular health and burning calories in a shorter timeframe. Common examples include sprinting, jumping, and short, intense intervals of cycling.

Benefits of Exercise

1. **Physical Health:**

    - Heart Health: Engaging in regular aerobic exercise strengthens the heart, enhances circulation, and lowers the risk of heart disease, high blood pressure, and stroke.

    - Muscle and Bone Health: Strength training improves muscle tone, increases bone density, and helps prevent conditions such as osteoporosis and muscle loss as you age.

- Weight Management: Exercise aids in calorie burning, supports metabolism, and contributes to maintaining a healthy weight.

- Improved Flexibility and Mobility: Stretching exercises enhance flexibility, decrease muscle stiffness, and boost overall mobility.

2. **Mental and Emotional Well-being:**

- Reduces Stress and Anxiety: Physical activity triggers the release of endorphins, which are natural chemicals that alleviate stress, anxiety, and depressive symptoms.

- Boosts Mood: Regular exercise promotes mental clarity, elevates self-esteem, and strengthens emotional resilience.

- Improves Sleep: Consistent physical activity can enhance sleep quality and assist with issues such as insomnia or restless sleep.

3. **Cognitive Benefits:**

- Improves Focus and Memory: Exercise increases blood flow to the brain, enhancing concentration, memory, and overall cognitive function.

- Delays Cognitive Decline: Regular physical activity may help lower the risk of age-related cognitive decline, including conditions like Alzheimer's disease.

4. **Increased Energy Levels:**

   - Routine exercise boosts stamina and reduces fatigue, leading to increased energy levels over time by enhancing cardiovascular efficiency and muscular endurance.

5. **Disease Prevention:**

   - Exercise lowers the risk of chronic conditions, such as type 2 diabetes, certain cancers, and metabolic syndrome, while also improving immune function.

Guidelines for Effective Exercise

- Frequency: Aim for at least 150 minutes of moderate aerobic activity or 75 minutes of vigorous activity weekly, along with muscle-strengthening exercises on two or more days.

- Consistency: The benefits of exercise are best realised through regular, consistent practice. Even small amounts of daily activity can accumulate to make a significant difference over time.

- Variety: Include a range of exercise types (aerobic, strength, flexibility) to ensure a balanced workout routine that targets all aspects of fitness.

- Rest and Recovery: Allow adequate time for rest between intense workouts to give your muscles a chance to recover, helping to prevent injury or burnout.

Examples of Exercise Routines

- Beginner: Engage in 30 minutes of brisk walking or light jogging, followed by 10 minutes of stretching, 3 to 5 days a week.

- Intermediate: Perform 45 minutes of a combination of cardio exercises (such as running or cycling) and strength training (including push-ups, squats, and light weights) 4 to 5 days a week.

- Advanced: Incorporate high-intensity interval training (HIIT) alongside strength training and mobility exercises like yoga, 5 to 6 days a week.

Understanding the significance of regular exercise is vital for maintaining both our physical health and mental well-being. Engaging in physical activity is not just about improving fitness; it plays a crucial role in enhancing our overall quality of life. When we exercise, our bodies and brains experience numerous positive changes. One of the most important aspects of exercise is its ability to provide us with increased energy levels. As we become more active, we boost our cardiovascular health, improve circulation, and enhance our stamina. This increased energy can lead to better performance in daily tasks, reduced fatigue, and an overall sense of vitality.

Moreover, exercise is essential for optimising cognitive function. Physical activity triggers the release of various neurotransmitters and hormones that positively influence our mood and emotional state. For instance, when we engage in exercise, our brains release

endorphins, often referred to as "feel-good" hormones. These chemicals contribute to a sense of euphoria, helping to elevate our mood and reduce the perception of pain. This natural high is one of the reasons people often feel a sense of accomplishment and happiness after a workout.

In addition to endorphins, our bodies produce **endocannabinoids** during exercise. These are neurotransmitters that also play a role in creating feelings of well-being and relaxation. They can help ease stress and promote a calmer state of mind, making physical activity a powerful tool for managing anxiety and enhancing mental health. Another important chemical released during exercise is **dopamine**, known as the "reward" neurotransmitter. Dopamine is crucial for motivation and pleasure, reinforcing the positive feelings associated with physical activity. It contributes to a sense of temporary gratification during and after exercise, encouraging individuals to stay active and maintain their fitness routines. This connection between exercise and dopamine can lead to a cycle of increased motivation and enjoyment, further promoting a healthy lifestyle.

Overall, the effects of regular exercise extend beyond physical fitness. By incorporating physical activity into our daily routines, we not only improve our physical health but also enhance our mental and emotional well-being. Regular exercise fosters a sense of vitality, boosts mood, and strengthens our resilience against stress and anxiety, making it a fundamental component of a balanced and healthy life.

The Impact of Exercise on Brain Health

Exercise has significant benefits for our brain, particularly in promoting **neuroplasticity**, which is the brain's ability to reorganise and create new neural connections. This is essential for learning and memory. When we engage in physical activity, it increases the flow of oxygen to the brain, which is crucial for maintaining cognitive functions and supporting overall mental health. Alongside this, exercise boosts the release of **serotonin**, a neurotransmitter linked to feelings of happiness and well-being. Higher serotonin levels contribute to a sustained positive mood and greater emotional stability. Thus, by incorporating regular exercise into our daily lives, we not only support our physical health but also enhance our mental and emotional well-being. Understanding how exercise affects the brain helps us appreciate its role as an essential part of a balanced and healthy lifestyle.

The 4-7-8 Breathing Technique

One effective method for improving sleep quality and managing anxiety is the **4-7-8 breathing technique**. This straightforward technique involves inhaling deeply through your nose for 4 seconds, holding your breath for 7 seconds, and then exhaling slowly through your mouth for 8 seconds. This intentional breathing pattern activates the **parasympathetic nervous system**, which helps induce a state of calm and relaxation. Practising this technique at night while lying in bed can help quiet your mind and promote the onset of sleep. Additionally, the 4-7-8 technique can be valuable during the day for managing stress and anxiety. By consciously engaging in this breathing exercise, you can lower your heart rate and blood pressure, reducing feelings of tension and stress. Regular practice may also help regulate **cortisol**, a hormone associated with the body's stress response. By keeping cortisol levels in check, you may experience better overall well-being and reduce the risk of long-term health issues related to chronic stress. Incorporating the 4-7-8 breathing technique into your daily routine can lead to significant improvements in both mental and physical health.

Surya Namaskara (Sun Salutation)

Starting your day with Surya Namaskara, or Sun Salutation, is an excellent practice. This dynamic sequence of yoga comprises 12 flowing postures or asanas, each coordinated with your breath. The practice is both meditative and energising, providing a comprehensive workout for your body. Regularly practising Surya Namaskara can improve flexibility, strength, and stamina. As you flow through the sequence, you'll find your muscles becoming more toned and your body increasingly flexible, benefiting your overall cardiovascular health. Furthermore, the advantages of Surya Namaskara extend beyond physical fitness. This sequence stimulates your nervous system, promotes muscle stretching and toning, and can assist with weight management. Research indicates that engaging in Surya Namaskara can bolster immune system function, enhance cognitive abilities, and support overall health and well-being. Incorporating this ancient practice into your daily routine can lead to greater vitality, balance, and inner peace. Surya Namaskara nourishes your body while soothing your mind, making it an essential component of a holistic approach to health and wellness.

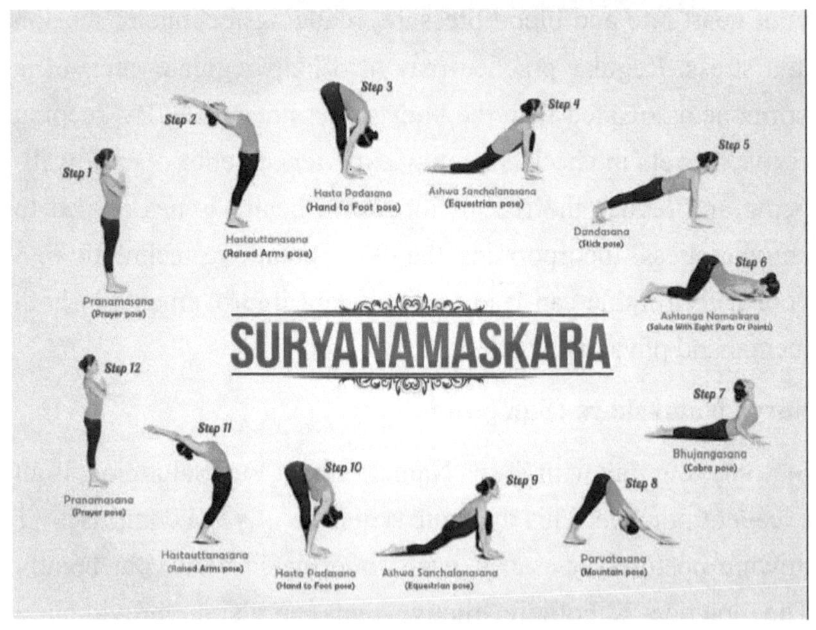

READING

Reading books offers numerous advantages that can help you grow personally and intellectually. By exploring different characters and stories, you better understand human nature and emotions. This is particularly useful in both your personal relationships and professional life. Throughout history, people have encountered and solved problems, many of which have been documented in books. These written works provide solutions that help others in the future. By reading, you can gain knowledge that might have taken years to accumulate, all within the span of a few hours.

Here are some of the major benefits that come from engaging with books:

- **Knowledge and Learning**: Books are excellent resources for gaining knowledge. They cover countless topics and provide valuable insights into a variety of subjects, helping you understand the world better.

- **Mental Stimulation**: Just as exercise keeps your body fit, reading stimulates your brain. It helps maintain mental sharpness and may even slow cognitive decline as you age. It also boosts memory, focus, and thinking skills.

- **Personal Growth and Improvement**: Reading introduces you to new ideas and perspectives, helping you challenge your current ways of thinking. It also provides motivation to develop better habits and can improve emotional intelligence.

- **Stress Relief and Relaxation**: Getting absorbed in a good book can help you unwind and forget the stress of daily life. It provides an escape, allowing your mind to relax and anxiety to reduce.

- **Creativity and Imagination**: Books, particularly fiction, stimulate your imagination. They transport you to different realities, encouraging creative thinking and expanding your imagination in everyday life.

- **Improved Focus and Concentration**: In today's fast-paced world, distractions are everywhere. Reading helps you slow down and focus more and can improve your attention span. This increased concentration can also make you more productive in other tasks.

- **Empathy Development**: By reading about the lives and experiences of others, especially from diverse backgrounds, you can develop empathy. Understanding different emotions and perspectives helps foster compassion for others.

- **Better Communication and Writing Skills**: Reading regularly can expand your vocabulary and improve grammar. This strengthens your ability to express thoughts clearly, both in writing and speaking.

- **Discipline and Consistency**: A regular reading habit helps develop discipline. Setting aside time to read daily builds self-discipline, which can improve time management and productivity.

- **Entertainment and Enjoyment**: Whether you enjoy fiction or non-fiction, books provide entertainment that often goes deeper than other forms of media, like TV. The immersive experience of reading is intellectually rewarding.

- **Improved Sleep**: Reading before bed can signal your brain that it's time to relax. Choosing a book over digital screens can lead to better sleep quality and help you wind down more effectively.

- **Lifelong Learning**: Books allow for continuous learning throughout life. They help you grow professionally and personally by providing endless opportunities for self-improvement and exploration of new hobbies or interests.

The Best Times to Read:

1. **Early Morning (Before or After Breakfast)**: Your mind is usually fresh in the morning, making it a great time to focus on thoughtful or reflective reading. This enhances your ability to remember what you've read and gives you a peaceful start to the day.

2. **Midday (During a Break or Lunch)**: Taking a break from work or daily tasks by reading can refresh your mind. It also offers a mental escape, helping reduce stress and leaving you feeling recharged.

3. **Afternoon (After Lunch)**: During the afternoon slump, light reading is a good way to relax without overexerting yourself. It helps re-energise your mind in a low-energy part of the day.

4. **Late Afternoon or Early Evening**: After you've completed your major tasks for the day, this time is perfect for reading at a more leisurely pace. It helps transition from work to relaxation.

5. **Before Bed**: Reading before bed is a great way to wind down. Non-fiction, motivational, or self-development paper books are ideal at night, as they can calm your mind and prepare you for sleep. Avoid stimulating content like thrillers, as these can make it harder to relax.

Personal Reading Routine:

- **Consistency**: The best reading time depends on your

schedule, but consistency is key. Dedicating 40 minutes to an hour each day—especially in the morning or before bed—can lead to personal growth over time.

- **Energy Levels**: Depending on your reading goals, choose times when you're most alert or relaxed. Mornings may be best for learning new things, while evenings are better suited for unwinding with less demanding material.

- **Book Type**: Choose the right book for the time of day. Non-fiction and self-improvement books are great for winding down, while educational content is best read when your mind is fresh in the morning.

Reading is essential for nourishing your mind, expanding your horizons, and offering opportunities for reflection and growth. Neglecting to read regularly can hinder mental stimulation and limit personal development.

THE VALUE OF WRITING

Incorporating writing into your daily routine can be a highly beneficial practice for several reasons. Here's a detailed explanation of its advantages:

1. Enhances Communication Skills

Writing regularly sharpens your ability to articulate thoughts clearly and effectively. As you practice, you learn to organise ideas and express them concisely, which can improve both your written and verbal communication skills.

2. Boosts Creativity

Daily writing fosters creativity by encouraging you to explore new ideas and perspectives. Whether it's through journaling, creative writing, or blogging, the act of writing allows you to experiment with language, style, and content, stimulating your creative thinking.

3. Improves Mental Clarity

Putting thoughts into words helps clarify your thinking. It allows you to process emotions, reflect on experiences, and understand complex situations better. Writing can serve as a mental detox, clearing cluttered thoughts and leading to greater insight.

4. Establishes a Routine

A dedicated writing routine cultivates discipline and consistency. Setting aside time each day to write can establish a productive habit, creating structure in your daily life. This routine can enhance focus and time management skills.

5. Serves as a Record of Growth

Daily writing provides a tangible record of your thoughts, ideas, and progress over time. Whether it's through a journal, a blog, or professional documentation, reviewing past entries can help you track personal growth and recognise patterns in your thinking.

6. Enhances Emotional Well-being

Writing can be a therapeutic outlet for emotions. It allows individuals to express feelings, cope with stress, and work through challenges. Journaling, in particular, has been linked to improved emotional health and resilience.

7. Encourages Lifelong Learning

Daily writing can inspire you to engage with new topics and continue learning. Researching subjects to write about or exploring different styles and genres can expand your knowledge and keep your mind engaged.

Making writing a daily practice is a valuable endeavour that can enhance communication skills, boost creativity, improve mental clarity, and contribute to emotional well-being. By dedicating time each day to writing, you can establish a routine that supports personal growth and lifelong learning, ultimately enriching your life in meaningful ways.

INTERMITTENT FASTING (IF)

Intermittent fasting (IF) is a straightforward and effective practice that enhances overall health. One of the most manageable methods is following a daily 12—to 14-hour fasting window, which allows the body time to rest, repair, and rejuvenate. A typical approach involves fasting from 8:00 PM to 8:00 AM, which naturally aligns with your sleep cycle. This method is easy to integrate into everyday life without significant disruptions.

How Intermittent Fasting Works

During the fasting period, your body isn't focused on digesting food. Instead, it redirects energy toward essential processes such as cellular repair, detoxification, and fat metabolism. As the body gets a break from food, insulin levels decrease, allowing fat stores to be used for energy. This mechanism supports weight management, stabilises blood sugar, and reduces the risk of chronic diseases. Intermittent fasting also encourages mindful eating. Because you have a defined eating window of 10 to 12 hours, you're less likely to snack continuously, giving your digestive system the rest it needs. Over time, this fosters improved digestion and more efficient nutrient absorption.

Benefits of a 12- to 14-Hour Fasting Window

1. **Improved Metabolism**: A 12—to 14-hour fasting period helps your body become more efficient at using stored fat for energy. This can assist with maintaining a healthy weight and lowering the risk of metabolic disorders like type 2 diabetes.

2. **Enhanced Digestion**: Giving your digestive system a regular break prevents it from becoming overworked, promotes better gut health, and reduces issues like bloating.

3. **Steady Energy Levels**: Fasting helps regulate blood sugar and promotes stable energy throughout the day. With the body's natural processes optimised during fasting, you may experience fewer energy dips and crashes.

4.. **Cellular Repair and Detoxification**: During fasting, the body activates autophagy, a process that cleans out damaged cells and regenerates healthier ones. This contributes to reduced inflammation, protection against disease, and potentially slowing down the ageing process.

5. **Mental Clarity**: Fasting supports brain function by minimising the body's energy needs for digestion. This frees up energy for better cognitive performance, enhancing focus and concentration.

6. **Ease of Adoption**: A 12- —to 14-hour fasting routine is one of the most accessible forms of intermittent fasting. Since much of the fasting happens during sleep, it is relatively easy to adopt without feeling deprived.

How to Implement Intermittent Fasting In One of The Simple Way

To incorporate intermittent fasting, aim to finish dinner by 8:00 PM and refrain from eating until 8:00 AM the next day. Avoid snacks or high-calorie drinks during the fasting period. Staying hydrated with water is critical. Herbal teas or black coffee are optional, as these won't break the fast but will keep you refreshed. If you're new to fasting, start with a 12-hour window, from 8:00 PM to 8:00 AM, and gradually extend it to 14 hours once your body adjusts. Listen to your body's signals and ensure your fasting routine feels manageable and comfortable over time.

Incorporating a 12 to 14-hour fasting window into your daily routine is a simple yet powerful way to boost your health. The benefits include improved digestion, better metabolism, mental clarity, and promoting cellular repair. Fasting between 8:00 PM and 8:00 AM allows your body time to rest, recover, and function optimally. This routine is an effective approach to improving long-term health and overall well-being.

The practice of fasting for one day each week is found in many cultures, health practices, and religious traditions. It typically involves voluntarily abstaining from food, or specific types of food, for 24 hours or a designated part of the day. This practice, often called "weekly fasting," is embraced for spiritual, cultural, and health-related purposes. In religious contexts, such as Islam, Christianity, Hinduism, and Buddhism, fasting is seen as a way to purify the soul, develop discipline, and promote mindfulness. From a health perspective, weekly fasting can improve digestion, boost metabolism, enhance mental clarity, and support cellular repair.

However, Intermittent fasting (IF) is a popular method where people fast for 12-16 hours daily or 24 hours once or twice a week. Some may adopt it as a regular habit. This approach can help manage weight, improve metabolism, and reduce inflammation. Other fasting types, like fruit or juice fasting, are used for detox and overall health. Fasting can benefit the body, mind, and spirit when practised correctly. However, if necessary, it's essential to seek medical advice before starting any fasting routine to ensure it's safe and suitable for your health needs

CREATING A BALANCED AND FULFILLING LIFESTYLE THROUGH GARDENING AND TREE PLANTING

Gardening and tree planting are practices that harmonise with the rhythms of nature, providing a powerful way to cultivate physical, mental, and environmental well-being. When integrated into daily routines, these activities promote personal health and contribute to a more sustainable and resilient planet. Both gardening and tree planting share core principles of care, patience, and responsibility, directly linking nurturing life and enhancing holistic health. Here's how both practices intersect and complement each other:

1. Physical Health and Activity

Both gardening and tree planting involve physical activities such as digging, lifting, and planting, which offer gentle exercise for the body. These activities improve cardiovascular health, strengthen muscles, and enhance flexibility. Engaging in these forms of movement outdoors also promotes the intake of fresh air and natural sunlight, which are essential for overall physical health. By making either or both practices a part of your routine, you actively support your body's fitness and endurance, making them excellent complementary practices.

2. Mental and Emotional Well-being

Gardening and tree planting have a calming and restorative effect on the mind, offering stress relief and a sense of fulfilment. The tactile nature of working with soil and plants helps individuals feel more grounded and connected to the earth, reducing anxiety and promoting mindfulness. While gardening provides immediate satisfaction as you see flowers bloom or herbs grow, tree planting is a long-term endeavour that teaches patience and perseverance. Watching a tree grow over months and years serves as a powerful reminder of the gradual yet rewarding nature of personal growth, making these practices both therapeutic and enriching.

3. Environmental Contribution and Sustainability

On a broader scale, gardening and tree planting contribute to environmental health by supporting biodiversity and reducing pollution. In gardening, growing a variety of plants can attract beneficial insects, promote soil health, and improve local ecosystems. Similarly, planting trees helps sequester carbon, improve air quality, and prevent soil erosion. When viewed together, these activities become acts of environmental stewardship, emphasising an individual's role in contributing to a greener planet. A garden filled with trees, shrubs, and flowering plants can serve as a microcosm of a balanced ecosystem, showcasing how small efforts accumulate into significant environmental impact.

4. Personal Growth and Responsibility

Both gardening and tree planting require consistent care and attention, teaching valuable lessons in patience, responsibility, and the rewards of nurturing life. Whether tending to a garden on a daily basis or ensuring a sapling's healthy growth, these practices instil habits of dedication and mindfulness. By observing the natural cycles of growth and change, individuals learn to appreciate the slow and steady process of development, both in plants and in themselves.

5. Family and Community Bonding

Gardening and tree planting offer wonderful opportunities for family and community engagement. Both activities can be enjoyed with children, teaching them about nature and instilling values of environmental responsibility. When practised as a group activity, they foster a sense of collaboration and shared purpose, whether planting a garden at home or participating in a community tree-planting event. These activities thus extend beyond individual benefits, creating social bonds and encouraging collective action for a healthier environment.

6. Establishing a Daily Practice and Routine

Incorporating gardening and tree planting into one's daily, weekly, or monthly routine brings a sense of structure and purpose to the day. Regular gardening can involve simple tasks such as watering, pruning, or weeding, while tree planting may include choosing new locations or monitoring existing plantings. The consistent attention and effort required for these practices help build discipline and time management skills. Setting aside time each day to connect with nature, whether through gardening or tree planting, ensures a balanced lifestyle that integrates mental, physical, and environmental well-being.

Creating a Synergistic Practice

Incorporating both gardening and tree planting into your routine can create a synergistic approach to holistic health. While gardening provides immediate, tangible rewards through the cultivation of flowers and edible plants, tree planting offers a long-term investment in the future as tree planting helps future generations by enhancing air quality, reducing carbon dioxide levels, and mitigating climate change. It also fosters biodiversity, creates healthier ecosystems, and provides natural resources like fruits and shade. These efforts ensure a cleaner, greener environment, promoting a sustainable legacy for the well-being of future communities. Together, these practices can be a profound reminder of life's cycles and our role in nurturing and sustaining them.

Overall, adopting gardening and tree planting as regular practices can transform not only the individual's lifestyle but also the environment around them. By caring for plants and trees, we engage in a reciprocal relationship with nature—one that nurtures both personal well-being and planetary health. The interconnected benefits of these practices make them powerful tools for cultivating a balanced and fulfilling lifestyle.

SUMMARY OF GARDENING AND TREE PLANTING FOR A BALANCED LIFESTYLE

1. **Physical Health**: Both activities offer light exercise, improve flexibility, and increase Vitamin D levels.

2. **Mental Well-being**: Reduce stress, boost mindfulness, and foster a sense of calm.

3. **Environmental Impact**: Enhance biodiversity, improve air quality, and contribute to sustainability.

4. **Personal Growth**: Teach patience, responsibility, and dedication.

5. **Family Bonding**: Serve as engaging, educational activities for all ages.

6. **Routine and Purpose**: Establish daily structure and provide a fulfilling sense of achievement.

THE IMPORTANCE OF SILENCE

•	**Embracing Morning Silence:** Cultivating a practice of silence in the tranquil moments of the morning, immediately upon awakening, can serve as a powerful tool to ready the mind for the day ahead. This serene interlude aids in centring thoughts, fostering mindfulness and sharpening focus. It is a practice highly esteemed in spiritual disciplines, meditation regimens, and self-improvement rituals. By embracing silence in the morning, one can alleviate anxiety, enhance mental clarity, and lay the groundwork for a more productive day.

•	**Midday Moments of Silence:** Carving out time for silence in the heart of the day, particularly after periods of intense work or activity, offers a valuable mental reset. It affords the brain an opportunity to replenish its resources and effectively manage stress. This practice might entail simply sitting quietly for a few minutes, engaging in meditation, or mindfully savouring a meal. Research indicates that interludes of silence enhance cognitive function and creativity, thereby positively influencing performance and decision-making.

•	**Evening Embrace of Silence:** Integrating moments of silence before bedtime has the profound effect of soothing the mind and readying the body for rest. This practice facilitates the transition from the day's clamour and tension, fostering relaxation and elevating the quality of sleep. Creating a tranquil environment before sleep bolsters the capacity to drift into slumber more swiftly and diminishes restlessness during the night.

Benefits of Daily Silence

The absence of noise has been shown to have a positive impact on mental health by reducing stress and anxiety. Studies have found that silence can effectively lower cortisol levels, which is the hormone responsible for stress. This can lead to a calmer state of mind and help individuals better manage their emotional reactions, ultimately improving their overall mental well-being. Furthermore, incorporating regular silent breaks into one's routine has been found to enhance focus and productivity. This practice can increase attention span and concentration, allowing the brain to process information more effectively and improving problem-solving skills. In addition, silence has been linked to boosting creativity. It activates areas of the brain associated with creativity and insight, enabling individuals to think more freely and come up with new ideas. Finally, practising silence allows individuals to reflect on their emotions and thoughts, leading to better emotional regulation and self-awareness. This can ultimately contribute to improved mental and emotional well-being.

Practising daily moments of silence, even for just a few minutes, can have numerous benefits for mental and physical well-being.

INTEGRATING ACTS OF KINDNESS, FORGIVENESS AND ACCEPTANCE

Implementing acts of giving and service into our daily routine is more straightforward than it seems and can profoundly impact us and others. This habit begins with a shift in mindset—seeing every interaction and moment as an opportunity to add value, show kindness, or brighten someone's day. Whether it's offering your time, skills, or a kind word, each small effort matters.

1. **Start Your Day with Intention**: Begin each morning by setting a clear intention to be helpful. This could involve listening more attentively, showing patience, or assisting a family member or colleague without being asked.

2. **Create a Daily Giving Practice**: Choose one small act of kindness to include in your routine, like buying a meal for someone in need, sharing your knowledge, or volunteering a few minutes to help a neighbour.

3. **Integrate Service into Routine Activities**: Service doesn't have to be separate from your regular schedule. Offer a word of encouragement, pick up litter during a walk, or teach something new to a friend or family member.

4. **Express Gratitude and Recognition**: Serve others by acknowledging their efforts with a simple thank-you note or verbal appreciation, which can significantly brighten someone's day.

5. **Lead by Example in the Family**: Involve family

members, especially children, in small acts of giving, like helping an elderly neighbour, cooking a meal for a friend, or planting trees to give back to nature. This strengthens family bonds and instils a habit of service early on.

6. **Use Your Talents and Skills**: Consider how your strengths can benefit others. If you're good at cooking, prepare a meal for someone in need. If you're tech-savvy, help others with digital tools.

7. **Reflect and Plan**: At the end of each day, reflect on how your actions contributed positively and set new goals for the next day. This reflection will make service a natural part of your routine.

When we give selflessly, the universe often returns our kindness in surprising ways, frequently multiplying the impact. This principle is not limited to material rewards; it embodies a deeper concept of reciprocity. By offering love, support, or resources, we create a positive flow of energy that attracts good outcomes back into our lives, often in unexpected forms.

For instance, extending help to someone might not only strengthen relationships but could also unlock new opportunities, enhance our well-being, and foster a sense of inner fulfilment, making the act of giving truly enriching. Incorporating service into our daily lives creates a cycle of giving that benefits others and nurtures our well-being. It strengthens communities, teaches humility and gratitude, and provides a profound sense of satisfaction. Ultimately, giving and serving regularly make us more empathetic, grounded, and purposeful, enriching our lives with deeper joy and meaning.

INTEGRATING FORGIVENESS AND ACCEPTANCE

Incorporating forgiveness and acceptance into our daily lives is essential for personal growth and emotional well-being. These practices require a conscious effort to shift our mindset, allowing us to release negative emotions and cultivate a more peaceful existence.

Here are some effective ways to implement forgiveness and acceptance into your routine:

1. **Practice Self-Compassion:** Begin by forgiving yourself for past mistakes and accepting that everyone is human. Recognise that making errors is a part of the learning process, and treat yourself with the same kindness you would extend to a friend. This self-acceptance lays the foundation for forgiving others.

2. **Identify and Acknowledge Grievances:** Take time to reflect on any grudges or resentments you hold against others. Writing them down can help you articulate your feelings. Acknowledging these emotions is the first step toward letting them go.

3. **Cultivate Empathy:** Try to understand the perspectives of those who have hurt you. Consider their circumstances

and motivations. This empathy can help soften your feelings of anger or resentment, making it easier to forgive.

4. **Set Boundaries:** While forgiveness is essential, it's equally important to set boundaries with those who have wronged you. Accepting that you can forgive someone without allowing them back into your life can protect your emotional health.

5. **Practice Mindfulness:** Engage in mindfulness exercises to help you stay present and focused. This practice can provide clarity and reduce the weight of negative emotions, allowing you to approach forgiveness with a clear mind.

6. **Express Your Feelings:** If appropriate, communicate your feelings to the person who hurt you. This could involve a heartfelt conversation or even a letter expressing your thoughts and emotions without placing blame. This act of expression can facilitate healing and foster understanding.

7. **Let Go of Control:** You cannot change the past or control others' actions. Embrace that moving forward requires releasing your grip on what has already happened. Acceptance is a powerful tool for freeing yourself from emotional burdens.

8. **Engage in Reflective Practices:** At the end of each day, reflect on your experiences with forgiveness and acceptance. Consider how these practices impacted your emotional state and relationships. This reflection can

help you identify areas for growth and reinforce your commitment to these values.

Incorporating forgiveness and acceptance into our daily lives is transformative. These practices foster emotional resilience, improve relationships, and enhance overall well-being. They allow us to move beyond anger and resentment, promoting peace and positivity. By embracing forgiveness and acceptance, we cultivate a more compassionate and harmonious existence for ourselves and those around us, leading to more profound joy and fulfilment.

THE TRANSFORMATIVE POWER OF MUSIC

Music plays a vital role in enhancing our daily routines and overall well-being. Its influence extends beyond mere enjoyment; it serves as a powerful tool for relaxation, focus, and motivation. Listening to music can trigger the release of dopamine, the "feel-good" neurotransmitter, effectively reducing stress and anxiety levels.

Starting your day with soothing melodies can set a positive tone, helping you feel more energised and productive. Conversely, upbeat tracks can supercharge your workouts, pushing you to achieve more significant results while making exercise more enjoyable.

Music also improves concentration and memory, making it an ideal companion for studying or working. It creates an environment conducive to deep focus, allowing you to absorb information more effectively. Furthermore, playing calming tunes in the evening promotes better sleep by soothing the nervous system and preparing your mind for rest.

Additionally, music serves as a powerful medium for emotional expression, fostering creativity and providing an outlet for feelings. Incorporating music into your daily life—whether through active listening during activities or as a calming backdrop during tasks—adds richness to your experiences, transforms mundane moments into meaningful ones, and enhances your overall mental and emotional health. Embracing the transformative power of music can lead to a more harmonious, fulfilling life.

SUMMARY

1. **Affirmation:**
   - o Start your day by affirming positive thoughts and beliefs.
   - o Use statements that reinforce your goals and self-confidence.

2. **Gratitude:**
   - o Express appreciation for the good things in your life.
   - o Cultivate a mindset of thankfulness to promote emotional well-being.

3. **Imagination:**
   - o Tap into your creative mind to envision new possibilities.
   - o Use imagination to explore ideas and plan your day creatively.

4. **Visualisation:**

   o Picture your goals and aspirations vividly.

   o Create a mental image of your desired outcomes to boost motivation.

5. **Vision Board:**

   o Compile images and words that represent your dreams and goals.

   o Use the board as a daily reminder to stay focused on long-term ambitions.

6. **Exercise:**

   o Engage in physical activity to energise your body and mind.

   o Choose exercises like yoga, stretching, or brisk walking for better stamina and health.

7. **Reading & the value of writing:**

   o Dedicate time to read books or articles that inspire or educate.

   o Enhance knowledge and stimulate mental growth.

   o Daily writing boosts communication, creativity, and emotional well-being while supporting personal growth. It establishes a productive routine for lifelong learning

8. **Intermittent Fasting:**

   o Implement a controlled eating pattern to optimise metabolic health.

   o Allows the body to reset and improve energy levels.

9. **Creating a Balanced and Fulfilling Lifestyle Through Gardening and Tree Planting:**

o Participate in gardening or tree planting to connect with nature.

o Promotes relaxation, environmental awareness, and sustainable living.

10. **The Importance of Silence:**

o Include moments of silence to reduce stress and improve focus.

o Helps cultivate mindfulness, self-reflection, and inner peace.

11. **Integrating Acts of Kindness, Forgiveness and Acceptance:**

o Regularly perform small acts of kindness, such as helping others, to foster a positive mindset and create a ripple effect of goodwill in your community.

o Embrace forgiveness and acceptance to release negative emotions and promote emotional resilience, enhancing personal growth and relationships.

o Reflect daily on your acts of kindness and experiences with forgiveness, allowing for growth and reinforcing the importance of these practices in your life.

12. **The Transformative Power of Music:**

o Music can lower anxiety and improve mood, creating a positive atmosphere and a sense of calm.

o Listening to music boosts concentration and productivity, making tasks more enjoyable while enriching our daily experiences.

Chapter

05

Evening Rituals

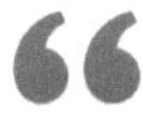

One cannot think, love, or sleep well if one has not dined well.

- Virginia Woolf

EVENING NOURISHMENT

As mentioned in the earlier chapter, this will follow. It is best to have dinner at least 2 - 3 hours before bedtime so your body can digest the food before you sleep. Dinner is typically eaten between 6:00 PM and 8:00 PM, but this timing can vary based on cultural norms and individual preferences.

Why Having an Early Dinner is Good for Health

Eating dinner early is a tradition and a habit that brings many health advantages. When you have your last meal of the day on time, it syncs well with your body's natural cycles, giving you many benefits that can improve your overall health and lifestyle.

• Better Digestion

When you eat early, your body has enough time to break down the food before you sleep. This can prevent problems like acidity, bloating, and indigestion. By giving your stomach enough time to digest, your body can absorb nutrients properly. This helps avoid uncomfortable issues like heartburn and keeps your digestive system healthy.

• **Improves Sleep**

Eating late can disturb your sleep because your body is still busy digesting the food when you are trying to rest. Having dinner early means your body finishes digesting before you go to bed, helping you sleep peacefully through the night. This leads to better, deeper sleep, which is important for your health.

• **Helps in Weight Management**

Eating late at night can lead to weight gain, as your body stores the extra calories when you are inactive. When you eat earlier, your body burns calories more efficiently because your metabolism works better during the daytime. By avoiding late-night snacks and overeating, an early dinner helps you control your weight better.

• **Controls Blood Sugar Levels**

Eating dinner late, especially a meal rich in carbohydrates, can spike your blood sugar levels. This is particularly dangerous for people with diabetes or insulin resistance. Eating an early dinner helps keep your blood sugar in control, reducing the risk of sudden insulin spikes and supporting better overall metabolism.

• **Boosts Energy**

When your body finishes digestion early, you wake up refreshed and full of energy. Early dinners ensure that the digestive system is not overworked overnight, making you feel more awake and energised the next morning, which sets a positive tone for the day.

- **Supports Intermittent Fasting**

Having dinner early naturally extends the time gap between dinner and breakfast, promoting intermittent fasting. This long gap helps in improving digestion, speeding up metabolism, and burning fat. These are essential for better health and can even aid in weight loss.

- **Syncs with Your Body Clock (Circadian Rhythm)**

Our body follows a natural cycle known as the circadian rhythm, which regulates many functions, including digestion. Eating earlier works well with this body clock and helps your body function at its best. It improves how your body processes food and helps maintain good health in the long run.

- **Prevents Chronic Diseases**

Studies show that eating late can increase the risk of developing serious health issues like obesity, diabetes, and heart disease. Eating dinner earlier eases the burden on your body's metabolism and digestive system. This, in turn, may lower the chances of developing lifestyle diseases such as type 2 diabetes or cardiovascular problems.

Ideal Time for Early Dinner

It is generally recommended to have dinner at least 2-3 hours before bedtime to allow for proper digestion and to avoid discomfort while sleeping. Ideally, dinner should be consumed around 6–8 PM if you typically go to bed around 9–10 PM. This schedule can help promote better sleep and overall digestive health.

Enjoying an early dinner can improve your overall well-being by helping you feel healthier and more energetic and supporting your long-term wellness goals. An early dinner gives your body more time to digest the food before bedtime, leading to better sleep and improved digestion. Additionally, it can help regulate your metabolism and prevent late-night snacking, which can positively impact your weight management efforts.

It can be tough for some people to shift to an earlier dinner time, but with gradual adjustments, it becomes easier. Start by having dinner 30 minutes earlier for one week, then move it another 30 minutes earlier the following week. Keep practising this over time, and you'll find it easier to enjoy an early dinner. Many individuals might feel hungry before bedtime, and some may even wake up at night because of hunger. This gradual approach can help you break unhealthy dining habits, reduce nighttime hunger, and allow your body to adjust over time. Additionally, staying hydrated and choosing lighter meals in the evening can support this transition and enhance your overall well-being. Foods like salads, soups, and whole grains can help satisfy your hunger without causing discomfort at night.

Ancient & Tribal Community Eating Culture:

In ancient times, people's eating habits were significantly impacted by the changing seasons, food accessibility, societal norms, and religious customs. Meals were less frequent but more substantial, emphasising utilising locally sourced, fresh, or preserved ingredients. Over time, these traditions have transformed into the more defined meal schedules we adhere to today, featuring distinct breakfast, lunch, and dinner times and an expansive array of dietary options.

In numerous tribal communities across India, the evening meal holds excellent significance within daily routines, playing an integral role in cultural customs and fostering social connections. These tribal societies tend to synchronise their mealtimes with natural patterns, often partaking in dinner early in the evening, shortly after sunset, or even before sunset. This practice reflects their agricultural way of life, commencing the day at dawn and concluding activities with the sunset.

1. Meal Structure

- **Locally Sourced and Seasonal Foods**: Tribal communities rely on locally available, seasonal ingredients. Their dinners usually consist of **millet**, **rice**, **lentils**, and **wild vegetables**, often cooked simply yet flavourful. If available, meat or fish may be included, especially during festivals or special occasions.

- **Community Preparation**: Meals are often cooked communally, with family or village members contributing, fostering a strong sense of togetherness.

2. Cultural Practices During Dinner

- **Sitting on the Floor**: Many tribal groups follow the traditional practice of sitting on the floor while eating, a posture believed to aid digestion.

- **Eating with Hands**: Eating with hands is common, as it

is believed to connect one more closely with the food and foster mindfulness.

3. Cultural and Social Activities

- **Storytelling and Music**: After dinner, tribal families often gather for **storytelling**, **folk songs**, and **dance**. These cultural activities pass down traditions, share knowledge, and strengthen social bonds.

- **Dance and Festivals**: During festivals, dinners are communal, with tribal folk dances like the **Gond** or **Santhal dance** performed around a fire. Music, drumming, and chanting are central, creating a joyful atmosphere that turns meals into cultural celebrations.

4. Seasonal Celebrations

Tribal dinners are often connected to the harvest season, where the community comes together to celebrate with feasts. Meals during these times are larger and more elaborate, reflecting the community's gratitude for the harvest and the earth's bounty.

Overall, tribal dinners in India are not just about nourishment; they are about **community**, **tradition**, and **celebration** of cultural identity, often accompanied by music, dance, and shared joy.

Japanese Eating Culture

Japanese people usually have well-rounded evening meals with various dishes. They follow the **"ichiju-sansai" principle**: "one soup, three sides." The **"ichiju-sansai" principle** in Japanese cuisine emphasises **variety** over **quantity**. The idea is to offer a well-balanced meal with various small, nutritious dishes rather than serving large portions.

- **"Ichiju"** means "one soup," typically miso soup.

- **"Sansai"** means "three sides," which includes grilled fish or meat, vegetables, and pickles.

These smaller, more diverse dishes are designed to provide a well-rounded intake of essential nutrients while ensuring that portions remain modest. This approach aims to deliver a satisfying dining experience without the risk of overheating, emphasising both health and mindfulness. Dinner is typically consumed early, usually between 6–8 PM, and centred around light and nutritious fare. In Japanese culture, there is a widely practised principle of eating until you are 80% full, known as **"Hara Hachi Bu,"** which originated in the Okinawan region but has significantly impacted broader Japanese dietary customs. Rather than striving to eat until complete, the focus is on maintaining moderation and balance. Meals traditionally comprise smaller, varied portions featuring various flavours and nutrients, as exemplified by the "ichiju-sansai" principle. This approach allows for a gratifying dining experience without the risk of excessive consumption.

Popular dinner choices in Japan include curry rice, ramen, and sushi, with each dish being enjoyed in different contexts. Curry rice is typically served as a home-cooked meal, ramen is often eaten at casual dining establishments, and sushi is usually reserved for special occasions or dining out. Traditional Japanese dining customs emphasise eating slowly and mindfully, especially when meals are shared with family. Meals are not only about nourishment but also about connection and gratitude. Green tea is a common beverage during meals, while sake and beer are typically enjoyed in social settings. Japanese cuisine prioritises balanced nutrition, using seasonal ingredients and low-fat cooking methods like steaming, grilling, and boiling.

Mindfulness during meals is deeply ingrained in Japanese culture. Before eating, it is customary to say **"Itadakimasu,"** a phrase expressing gratitude for the food, its preparation, and the life it represents. This reflects a mindful approach to dining, where meals are savoured slowly to enhance digestion and increase awareness of flavours and textures. While modern urban life may lead to faster meals at times, the principles of gratitude and mindfulness remain central to Japanese eating habits, reinforcing a deep cultural connection to the food and its origins.

Respect for seasonal ingredients is fundamental in Japanese cuisine, with food presentation regarded as an art form. The careful selection and arrangement of ingredients not only enhance the flavour but also reflect an appreciation for nature and the changing seasons. After finishing a meal, it is customary to say **"Gochisousama deshita,"** expressing gratitude to everyone involved in the meal's preparation. This mindful conclusion to the dining experience fosters appreciation for the effort, time, and care put into making and serving the food, reinforcing the values of respect and gratitude in Japanese culinary culture.

Portion Control Eating

Portion control is a mindful and intentional approach to selecting and consuming a balanced and nutritious serving size of a specific

food. It ensures that the body receives essential nutrients without excess intake. Portion control yields many benefits that positively impact overall health and well-being. **Portion control eating can be followed for your entire eating schedule.**

"Portion control plays a crucial role in managing weight by allowing individuals to keep track of their calorie intake, thus enabling them to achieve and maintain a healthy weight. It also helps prevent overeating by encouraging individuals to pay attention to their body's hunger and fullness cues. Additionally, smaller meals can ease digestion, reducing discomfort and bloating. Furthermore, practising portion control promotes a more mindful approach to eating, leading to a more balanced intake of essential nutrients. It also enhances awareness of portion sizes, empowering individuals to make more informed food choices and develop healthier dietary habits.

Moreover, controlled portions can significantly impact blood sugar levels, particularly beneficial for those with diabetes or insulin sensitivity. Consuming balanced portions can lead to feeling satisfied without being overly full, fostering a healthier relationship with food. Furthermore, portion control can decrease food waste and promote efficient meal planning. Incorporating mindful portion control practices can enhance overall well-being and lead to a healthier lifestyle."

Portion Control Eating & Hara Hachi Bu

Portion control eating and Hara Hachi Bu are related concepts but differ in their approach. Portion control focuses on regulating the amount of food consumed by measuring serving sizes to manage caloric intake and prevent overeating. It involves specific guidelines for how much food to eat at each meal. In contrast, Hara Hachi Bu, an Okinawan practice, encourages eating until you are about 80% full, promoting mindfulness and self-awareness rather than strict measurements. While both aim to prevent overeating and support health, portion control is more structured, while Hara Hachi Bu emphasises intuitive eating based on bodily cues.

Distractions while Eating Dinner

Engaging in distractions such as watching TV, using mobile devices, or reading while eating dinner can affect our eating habits and overall well-being.:

- Reduced awareness of portion sizes, potentially leading to overeating

- Diminished enjoyment and appreciation of the food being consumed

- Impaired digestion due to a lack of focus on chewing and mindful eating habits

- Disrupted communication and bonding among individuals sharing the meal

- Increased likelihood of consuming unhealthy or processed foods due to decreased attention to food choices.

Disinterest in Eating Dinner

To combat disinterest in having dinner and food boredom, you can try the following strategies with confidence:

1. **Introduce Variety**: Experiment with new recipes, cuisines, or ingredients to make meals more exciting and enjoyable. Trying different cooking methods or spices can change the experience of familiar dishes.

2. **Meal Planning**: Plan meals in advance to avoid repetitive eating. Incorporate a range of vegetables, proteins, and grains to ensure variety in taste and nutrition.

3. **Make Mealtime Enjoyable**: Create a pleasant dining atmosphere by setting the table nicely, eating with family or friends, or even playing soft music. This can make dinner feel more like an event rather than a routine.

4. **Smaller, More Frequent Meals**: If large dinners are unappealing, try eating smaller meals throughout the day, ensuring they're balanced and satisfying.

5. **Engage in Mindful Eating**: Focus on the flavours, textures, and enjoyment of the food, avoiding distractions like TV or phones. Mindful eating can increase appreciation for the meal.

These steps can renew interest in food and make dinner a more enjoyable part of the day.

Meal Preparation

Balancing a consistent and timely dinner schedule can be difficult, especially with work commitments, social gatherings like parties, and weekend activities. However, achieving this balance is feasible with strategic scheduling and meal preparation.

1. Plan Ahead

Prepare meals in advance or choose quick, healthy options to save time. Meal prepping or having easy-to-make dishes like salads or soups can help you stick to an early dinner, even after a busy day.

2. Set a Consistent Time

Aim to have dinner between **6 and 8** PM. Setting a routine helps your body adjust to early eating, promoting better digestion and sleep.

3. Healthy Choices at Parties

If you are at a party, choose lighter, healthier options or eat a small meal before attending. Avoid heavy, late-night eating, and try to finish eating at least **2-3 hours before bed**.

4. Mindful Eating

No matter how busy you are, eat slowly and mindfully. This helps digestion and allows you to enjoy your food, even during a hectic schedule.

5. Balance Social and Work Commitments

If work or social events push dinner later, aim for smaller portions or lighter meals at night to avoid feeling too full before sleep. Making small changes and prioritising mealtimes allows you to maintain a balanced and healthier dinner routine even with a busy lifestyle.

Choosing light, balanced, and nutrient-rich meals is best for easy digestion during dinner. Here are some suggestions:

- **Lean Proteins**: Choose easily digestible proteins like fish, chicken, and turkey or plant-based proteins such as tofu or lentils. Avoid heavy, fatty meats that can be harder to digest.

- **Cooked Vegetables**: Steamed or sautéed vegetables like spinach, zucchini, carrots, or green beans are easier on the stomach than raw ones. They provide essential nutrients without causing bloating.

- **Whole Grains**: Brown rice, quinoa, or whole wheat bread are good sources of fibre and aid digestion. Avoid refined carbs, which can be heavy and slow down digestion.

- **Healthy Fats**: Use small amounts of healthy fats like olive oil or avocado, which promote digestion and satiety without being too heavy.

- **Light Soups or Broths**: Broth-based soups or clear vegetable soups are gentle on the stomach, hydrating, and easy to digest.

- **Herbal Teas**: Post-dinner herbal teas like ginger or peppermint tea can help soothe digestion and prevent discomfort.

- **Rice and Lentils (Dal)**: A bowl of rice with lightly spiced lentils provides a balanced meal with protein, fibre, and carbohydrates, making it easy to digest and fill.

- **Roti with Vegetables**: Whole wheat rotis (flatbread) paired with cooked vegetables like spinach, pumpkin, or carrots offer a light, nutritious meal that is gentle on the stomach.

- **Khichdi**: A one-pot meal of rice and lentils cooked with minimal spices is easy to prepare, soothing for digestion, and an everyday staple in rural areas.

- **Millet (Ragi, Jowar, Bajra)**: Millets are light, nutrient-rich grains available in rural areas. Combined with curd or simple vegetable dishes, they provide a healthy, easily digestible meal.

- **Curd and Rice**: The simple yet satisfying combination of steamed rice and freshly prepared curd (yogurt) is renowned for its ability to cool the body and soothe the palate. gentle effect on the stomach and its ability to aid digestion. However, it may not be suitable for everyone, as consuming curd in the evening may not be advisable for some individuals.

- **Vegetable Soup**: A simple soup made with locally available vegetables can be light and hydrating, promoting easy digestion.

- **Fruits & Vegetables**: For a wholesome and easily digestible dinner option, choose light fruits like papaya, watermelon, and bananas. Pair them with cooked vegetables like sweet potatoes, spinach, or steamed broccoli for added fibre and nutrients. This combination is gentle on the stomach and keeps you satisfied.

Note: Food is a deeply personal choice that varies from person to person based on individual preferences. However, it is crucial to prioritise balanced nutrition to support overall well-being. It's always advisable to align your diet with your body's specific needs and your unique body type. Following a diet that is tailored to your individual Prakriti can significantly enhance your lifestyle and increase your overall happiness, contributing to a healthy and prolonged life.

It's essential that your dietary choices do not impose excessive constraints or burdens on your daily life; instead, they should feel effortless and natural, almost like following a "no-diet" approach. Additionally, food should be nourishing and enjoyable, focusing on delicious, appetising, and easily digestible options.

Wasting food and discarding food have negative consequences for several reasons

- Environmental Impact: Food waste produces landfill methane emissions, a potent greenhouse gas. It also squanders precious resources such as water, energy, and labour used in food production.

- Economic Costs: Wasting food results in financial losses for households and businesses, straining personal budgets and increasing food prices.

- Ethical Concerns: Food waste is particularly concerning in a world where many people face food insecurity, underscoring the imbalance between food abundance and distribution.

- Resource Inefficiency: Discarding food means that the

resources utilised to grow, transport, and prepare it are wasted when they could have been used more efficiently.

- Reducing food waste requires better planning, appropriate storage, and creative utilisation of leftovers to ensure that resources are utilised wisely and ethically.

To minimise food waste and prevent the disposal of food, consider employing the following approaches

- Plan and Prepare: Create a meal plan and shopping list to purchase only necessary items. Additionally, adopt a first-in, first-out system for pantry and fridge items to utilise older products first.

- Proper Storage: To prolong food's shelf life, ensure it is stored correctly. This involves using airtight containers, freezing leftovers, and maintaining perishable items at the appropriate temperatures.

- Portion Control: Serve smaller portions and encourage second helpings if necessary to prevent excessive food preparation.

- Creative Use of Leftovers: To decrease waste, transform leftovers into new dishes or incorporate them into future meals.

- Composting: Repurpose fruit and vegetable scraps by turning them into compost. This helps reduce waste sent to landfills and enriches soil for gardening purposes.

- Educate and Advocate: Increase awareness about food waste within your community and support policies or programs that minimise it.

EVENING ROUTINE & PRACTICES

Creating a balanced evening routine is essential for maintaining overall well-being and leading a more fulfilling and peaceful life. Your evening practices must address your mental, emotional, physical, and spiritual needs. Here's a detailed guide to help you establish the best evening routine that incorporates activities to nurture each aspect of your well-being.

1. Mental Well-Being Practices

In the evenings, allocating time for activities that help calm the mind and promote mental relaxation is important. This is essential for clearing the mind and getting ready for a peaceful night's sleep. This period is dedicated to learning how to unwind, manage emotions, and conclude the day on a positive note

Mindfulness Meditation and Deep Breathing:

- Mindfulness meditation involves sitting quietly, focusing on your breath, and letting go of any passing thoughts. Start by sitting in a comfortable posture with a straight back. Close your eyes and take slow, deep breaths. With each inhale, feel your body relaxing. As you exhale, release any tension. Focus on your breath, and gently bring your attention back to your breathing if your mind wanders. Just 10 minutes of this practice can calm your mind and reduce stress.

Visualisation Techniques:

- Another effective way to relax is through visualisation. Close your eyes and imagine a serene place—a calm beach, a quiet hilltop, or a lush green field. Try to picture every detail—the sound of birds, the gentle breeze, or the sun's warmth. Visualising such tranquil scenes can help reduce anxiety and improve mood.

Reflection and Journaling:

- Spend some time each evening thinking about your day. Sit peacefully and reflect on your emotions, interactions, and experiences. Note down your thoughts in a journal. Writing down both positive and challenging moments can help clear the mind. Include things you felt grateful for, as this practice boosts positivity and reduces stress.

Planning for Tomorrow:

- To ensure a smooth start to the next day, spend 5-10 minutes planning. Write down your tasks in order of priority. If you have appointments or meetings, add them to your planner or phone calendar. Doing this lets you sleep better, knowing you are prepared for the coming day.

Reading or Learning Something New:

- Before you go to bed, consider selecting a light book to read, preferably in paperback format. Look for non-fiction, self-development, motivational, or other similarly uplifting genres. Alternatively, you can listen to informative podcasts or read a short article that helps to calm your mind. It's best to avoid news or intense topics before bedtime. Choose content that promotes a sense of calm, positivity, or knowledge to help you end the day on a good note.

Suggestions: Make sure to focus on calming topics. Try to stay away from work-related or problem-solving material, as it may keep your mind too engaged to relax properly. Avoid reading newspapers, articles with negative information, scary or horror content, and anything disturbing your peace of mind.

2. Emotional Well-Being Practices

Emotional health is just as important as mental and physical health. How you feel in the evening affects how well you sleep and your emotional stability for the next day.

Gratitude Practice:

- Think about three good things that happened during the day, no matter how small. It could be a pleasant conversation, a meal you enjoyed, or just the fact that you completed a challenging task. Write these in a gratitude journal or say them aloud. This practice shifts focus from negative to positive experiences, promoting emotional resilience.

Emotional Check-In:

- Spend a minute observing your emotions without judgment. Ask yourself, "What am I feeling right now?" Name the emotion (e.g., "I feel content," "I feel overwhelmed"). Simply acknowledging your feelings helps you manage them better.

Connecting with Loved Ones:

- After a busy day, connect with your family. Share stories, talk about your day, or even enjoy a light-hearted conversation.

If you live alone, call a friend or family member. These interactions provide emotional support and reinforce positive relationships.

Suggestions: Avoid discussing serious matters before bed. Stick to positive and comforting topics that enhance bonding.

3. Physical Well-Being Practices

Light physical activities help release built-up tension, making it easier to sleep. The focus should be on gentle movements that relax your muscles.

Gentle Stretching or Yoga:

- Perform simple stretches like shoulder rolls, neck stretches, and back twists. Include yoga poses such as child's pose or seated forward bend. Begin with a few deep breaths to centre yourself. These stretches loosen muscles and relieve stiffness accumulated throughout the day, easing physical stress.

- **Light Walk After Dinner:**

- Walking 15-20 minutes after dinner can aid digestion and improve circulation. It's even more effective if you walk outdoors. The fresh air and rhythmic movement clear your mind, leaving you relaxed.

Soothing Bath or Shower:

- A warm shower or bath with a few drops of essential oils like lavender can do wonders for releasing muscle tension. Lavender and chamomile are known for their relaxing properties, which can induce a sense of calm. Add a handful of bath salts to relax muscles and promote a positive mood.

Suggestions: Intense physical activities should be avoided close to bedtime, as they may increase energy levels, making it harder to fall asleep.

4. Spiritual Well-Being Practices

These practices can vary depending on your beliefs. They aim to promote inner peace, purpose, and relaxation.

Meditation for Spiritual Grounding:

- Sit quietly in a dimly lit room. Close your eyes and focus on your breath. Slowly breathe in and out, concentrating on each inhale and exhale. If thoughts arise, let them pass without getting attached. This practice helps you feel grounded and peaceful.

Prayer or Spiritual Reading:

- If you practice a religion, evening prayer or reading from a spiritual text can be deeply calming. If not, spend a few minutes reflecting on your values and what brings you peace. Some find comfort in reading wisdom literature, poetry, or philosophical texts that align with their beliefs.

Deep Breathing Exercise (4-7-8 Method):

- Find a comfortable position, either sitting or lying on your bed. You can place one hand on your chest and the other on your belly to become more aware of your breathing, but this is optional. Inhale deeply through your nose for 4 seconds, hold your breath for 7 seconds, and then exhale slowly through your mouth for 8 seconds. Repeat this breathing pattern 4 to 5 times. This exercise helps calm the nervous system, alleviates anxiety, and prepares your body for rest.

Suggestions: Create a quiet, peaceful environment using dim lighting or candles to make your space feel more serene and comforting.

5. Sleep Preparation and Routine

A proper sleep routine is essential for good health. The focus should be on maintaining a consistent schedule and creating a relaxing atmosphere.

Regular Bedtime Routine:

- Aim to sleep at the same time each night to regulate your body's internal clock. This consistency will naturally make you feel sleepy around your set time and wake up refreshed.

Limit Screen Time:

- Avoid using phones and tablets or watching TV at least an hour before bed. Blue light from screens interferes with melatonin production, making sleeping difficult. Instead, engage in low-light activities like reading or listening to calming music.

Dim Lighting and Humidifiers:

- Use low, soft lighting in your bedroom before bed. Light a few scented candles or use a small lamp with warm light. Diffusing essential oils like lavender or sandalwood can create a relaxing atmosphere.

Herbal Teas:

- Drink herbal teas like chamomile or peppermint an hour before bed. They are known for their calming properties and can help the body prepare for rest.

Suggestions: Keep your bedroom environment calm and quiet. Use it only for sleeping, as this will help your mind associate the room with rest and relaxation.

SUMMARY

Eating dinner early, typically between 6:00 PM and 8:00 PM, aligns with the body's natural digestive rhythms and offers numerous health benefits. It aids in better digestion, improves sleep quality, supports weight management, and helps regulate blood sugar levels. Additionally, cultural practices, such as those seen in Japanese and various tribal communities, emphasise communal and mindful eating, highlighting the significance of meal timing and preparation. Strategies for maintaining an early dinner routine include meal planning, mindful eating, and portion control, which enhance overall well-being and reduce food waste. By fostering awareness around meal habits and making informed choices, individuals can contribute to healthier lifestyles and a more sustainable food system.

- **Mental Well-Being Practices** like meditation, visualisation, and deep breathing are well-recognised methods for reducing stress and promoting relaxation. Journaling and planning for the next day are also proven strategies for enhancing mental clarity and reducing anxiety.

- **Emotional Well-Being Practices** such as gratitude journaling, emotional check-ins, and connecting with loved ones are universally acknowledged to support emotional resilience and a positive mindset.

- **Physical Well-Being Practices** like light stretching, walking after meals, and taking warm showers are recommended by health professionals to promote relaxation and improve sleep quality.

- **Spiritual Well-Being Practices** are presented in a neutral way to include practices like mindfulness meditation, prayer, and reading, focusing on peace and self-reflection, which is applicable regardless of specific beliefs.

- **Sleep Preparation and Routine** elements like maintaining a regular sleep schedule, reducing screen time, and creating a relaxing environment are supported by sleep research and recommendations from health institutions.

Best Practices for Better Sleep and Overall Well-being:

- Have a light dinner at least 2 hours before bedtime to aid digestion and prevent discomfort during the night.

- The optimal sleeping time is between 10 PM and 4 AM, which aligns with natural circadian rhythms and allows for restorative sleep.

- Determine the amount of sleep your body requires by paying attention to how you feel after different sleep durations and

consistently aim to meet that need.

- Sync with your circadian rhythm by exposing yourself to natural light during the day and minimising exposure to artificial light, especially in the evening.

- If you feel groggy upon waking up, consider taking short afternoon naps to rejuvenate without disrupting your nighttime sleep. Ideally, keep these naps to around 20-30 minutes for maximum benefits. However, maintaining a consistent nighttime sleep schedule is crucial for overall health

- Create a conducive sleep environment by keeping your bedroom dark and electronic devices, such as smartphones, at least 20-30 feet away from your bed after 9 PM to limit exposure to stimulating light and content.

- Visualise your goals before bedtime and program your subconscious mind to wake up at a specific time through positive affirmations and mental rehearsal.

- Maintain a well-balanced daily routine that includes time for work, leisure, exercise, and relaxation to promote overall physical and mental well-being.

Incorporate mindfulness, prayers, and meditation practices into your daily routine to manage stress, enhance self-awareness and emotional well-being, and promote better

Chapter

06(A)

Together in Routine

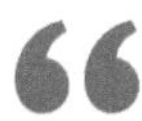

"Family is not an important thing; it's everything."
Michael J. Fox.

Establishing a structured and consistent family routine is crucial for the overall well-being of every family member. However, numerous challenges can arise when trying to establish such a routine. Waking up early, going to bed on time, sticking to regular mealtimes, following daily routines, and managing changes in schedule during weekends, long weekends, and holidays can all present difficulties. These challenges often result in increased stress, disrupted schedules, and unhealthy habits if they are not effectively addressed. In the upcoming comprehensive discussion, we will delve into these concerns, present effective approaches to address them, and provide suggestions for cultivating a peaceful and cohesive family environment, which is the ultimate goal of this routine and a key factor in improving overall well-being.

1. Challenges Associated with Early Morning Awakening

Maintaining a consistent bedtime routine is essential for ensuring that family members are able to wake up early feeling refreshed and well-rested. Irregular sleeping patterns can disrupt the body's internal clock, making waking up at the desired time difficult. Factors such as staying up late for work, social activities, or entertainment can contribute to sleep deprivation, reducing sleep quality and making it challenging to wake up early. However, it's not just about the physical aspect. A lack of motivation can also play a significant role in the difficulty of waking up early, especially for children and sometimes adults. Finding the motivation to rise and shine can be a struggle without a clear task or responsibility in the morning. Weekend habits can also impact wake-up times during the week. Sleeping on weekends can disrupt the body's natural rhythm, leading to inconsistency in wake-up times and making it difficult to get up early on weekdays.

How to Overcome

Establishing a consistent sleep schedule is crucial for the entire family's well-being. It's important to set fixed bedtimes for children and adults and stick to these bedtimes even on weekends. While it's acceptable to allow for some flexibility, such as a one-hour difference in bedtimes on weekends, it's essential to maintain a fairly consistent schedule.

Creating a positive morning routine can greatly impact the way everyone starts their day. Engaging in activities such as light exercise, yoga, family games, enjoying a family breakfast, or listening to uplifting music can motivate everyone to wake up early and start the day on a positive note.

Making gradual adjustments can be helpful for those who struggle with rising early. This involves shifting wake-up times earlier by 15 minutes each day or each week until the desired wake-up time is achieved. This approach is particularly effective for both children and adults who find it challenging to wake up early. It's important to ensure that the sleeping environment is conducive to proper rest. This includes creating a quiet, dark, and comfortable space for sleeping, which can enhance sleep quality and promote **the habit of rising early.**

2. Challenges in Maintaining a Consistent Sleep Schedule

Late-night screen time, such as using phones, watching TV, and using tablets, can overstimulate the brain and interfere with the body's natural bedtime routine. This can make it difficult to fall asleep and can delay the onset of sleep. Having irregular evening routines, including unplanned or disorganised evenings, can contribute to late dinners, scattered activities, and difficulties in winding down before bedtime. This can make it hard for the body and mind to relax and prepare for sleep.

Work and homework pressures can also contribute to late bedtimes, as parents may bring work home, and children may delay doing their homework, leading to later nights. Social distractions such as socialising, family gatherings, or staying out late can push bedtimes later than intended, disrupting the body's natural sleep-wake cycle.

How to Overcome

Remember to limit screen time before bedtime by ensuring that all electronic devices are turned off at least 60 minutes before bed. During this time, engage in relaxing activities such as reading a book, enjoying a calming conversation with family members, or participating in some of the evening practices outlined in this book. Additionally, it's helpful to establish a relaxing evening routine for the whole family. This may include gentle stretching exercises, reading, or spending quality time together for reflection. Using reminders or alarms can signal when it is time to start winding down in the evening, aiding both children and adults in transitioning from active evening activities to a restful state ready for sleep. Lastly, try to plan evening activities strategically, such as organising homework, work, and household chores earlier in the evening to avoid interfering with sleep.

3. Challenges with Meal Timing

The challenges of disorganised mealtimes are often a result of busy work schedules, conflicting after-school activities, a lack of coordination among family members, and other reasons. As a result, it's common for mealtimes to become irregular, leading to potential health issues. Skipping breakfast is a common occurrence due to the rushed nature of mornings. This can result in family members missing out on essential nutrients or resorting to unhealthy, quick snacks to curb their hunger. Late-night meals, especially after 8 PM, can disrupt the body's digestive processes and interfere with sleep quality. This can impact overall well-being and contribute to long-term health concerns. Frequent snacking between irregular meals can lead to overeating and unhealthy food choices. These snacks may be used as substitutes for proper meals, further exacerbating the issue of irregular eating patterns.

How to Overcome

Establishing regular mealtimes is crucial for the whole family's healthy eating routine. Setting fixed mealtimes for breakfast,

lunch, and dinner helps establish a sense of structure and consistency. This allows everyone to plan their day around these times, ensuring that they have time to eat and enjoy their meals.

Planning meals in advance can significantly reduce the stress and rush of preparing food during the week. Preparing meal plans or even pre-cooking meals over the weekend can save time and ensure that nutritious and delicious meals are ready to be enjoyed on time throughout the week. This proactive approach to meal preparation also minimises the chances of resorting to unhealthy or fast-food options due to time constraints. Avoiding eating late at night is important to promote good digestion and quality sleep. Finishing dinner at least two hours before bedtime allows the body to digest the food properly and promotes better sleep quality. Encouraging the family to adhere to this practice can positively affect their well-being.

Making breakfast a priority sets the tone for the day and provides much-needed energy. Preparing quick, healthy breakfast options the night before, such as overnight oats, pre-cut fruit, or yoghurt parfaits, ensures that everyone can start their day with a nutritious meal, even on busy mornings. By prioritising breakfast, everyone in the family can kick-start their day positively and maintain consistent energy levels throughout the morning.

4. Challenges Encountered in Daily Routines

Family members may face challenges in maintaining a consistent daily routine due to the unpredictability of work or school schedules or other reasons, resulting in increased stress and disorder. Furthermore, the lack of coordination between parents and children may lead to conflicts in managing time and responsibilities. Additionally, distractions and procrastination often disrupt household chores, work tasks, other reasons, and schoolwork due to a lack of organisation and focus.

How to Overcome

Organise a visual schedule encompassing every aspect of your family's daily routine. Assign specific times for waking up, preparing and enjoying meals, attending school or work, engaging in relaxation activities, and winding down for bedtime to ensure everyone stays on track. Delineate each family member's roles and responsibilities, encompassing homework assignments and household chores, and seamlessly integrate these tasks into the daily routine. Give particular emphasis to indispensable daily activities such as mealtimes, academic or professional obligations, and sufficient rest to maintain a consistent and harmonious schedule. Minimise household distractions, including excessive TV viewing, extended phone usage, and prolonged social media engagement during crucial periods to enhance everyone's concentration and productivity.

5. Challenges Related to Weekends, Extended Weekends, and Holidays

During weekends, holidays, and long weekends, it's common for families to shift their sleep schedule, staying up later and sleeping in. This deviation from their regular sleep routine often leads to difficulty reading to a typical schedule. Additionally, mealtimes tend to become less structured, with delayed eating and increased unhealthy snacking or overeating in the relaxed atmosphere. The lack of the usual work or school routine can make weekends and holidays feel chaotic, leading to disorganisation and stress. Furthermore, social events and family gatherings during holidays can further disrupt the normal daily routines.

How to Overcome

Maintaining a regular wake-up and bedtime schedule throughout the week, including weekends and holidays, with slight variations of up to 1 hour, is important, as consistent sleep patterns can positively impact overall well-being. Planning Ahead for Social Events: When scheduling social events, plan meals and bedtime to align with the family's routine to minimise disruptions and ensure everyone can enjoy the event while maintaining their regular schedule. Preparing for Weekdays: To smoothly transition from a long weekend or holiday back to the weekday routine, consider gradually adjusting sleep times and opting for lighter, nutritious meals to ease the transition and ensure everyone is well-rested and prepared for the upcoming week. Creating Flexible Holiday Routines: While weekends and holidays are typically more relaxed, it's beneficial to maintain a degree of structure by scheduling key activities such as meals and bedtime to provide a sense of stability while allowing for flexibility to indulge in enjoyable and relaxing experiences.

Gardening - A wonderful way for families to bond and learn together.

- **Shared Activity**: Engaging in gardening can be a wonderful way to unite family members and create lasting memories. It provides a platform for collaboration, communication, and skill-building, particularly beneficial for children, as they can cultivate an understanding and respect for the environment and gain a sense of ownership and accountability

- **Educational Value**: Gardening provides a wonderful opportunity for individuals of all ages to cultivate essential life skills, including patience, empathy, and a sense of environmental responsibility. By nurturing plants and fostering their growth, individuals can gain a deeper understanding of sustainability and develop a profound respect for the natural world.

Recommendations for Long-Term Success

- **Leading by Example**: As parents, we must model the behaviour we want our children to follow. This includes waking up on time, maintaining a healthy diet, and following a daily schedule.

- **Communicating with the Family**: Regular discussions should be held about what's working well and what isn't within the family routine. It's essential to involve everyone in adjusting routines when necessary.

- **Using Positive Reinforcement**: It's crucial to praise children and provide rewards when routines are followed successfully. This can be as simple as spending quality family time together or giving small rewards for consistency.

- **Being Flexible When Needed**: While structure is important, it's also essential to remain flexible, particularly during holidays or weekends. The goal is to find a balance between routine and relaxation.

- **Incorporating Relaxing Activities**: Scheduling family relaxation time ensures everyone feels refreshed. Activities such as walking, playing indoor games, practising meditation, or reading together in the evenings can be included.

- **Get the Family Involved**: Encourage family members to join, turning gardening into a shared activity that can strengthen bonds.

- **Healthy Habits for All**: Teaching children the importance of balance, sleep, and healthy eating is vital. Involving them in meal preparation and decision-making for daily routines can help instil these healthy habits from a young age."

In the earlier generations, children spent hours enjoying the great outdoors, which significantly contributed to their overall health and well-being. Whether through imaginative play, exploration of the natural world, or interaction with peers, outdoor activities profoundly impacted their physical, mental, and emotional development. The freedom to roam and play in natural settings provided ample opportunities for creativity, problem-solving, and hands-on learning, fostering a holistic connection between their minds, bodies, and emotions. Now, let's delve into a comprehensive comparison of the myriad benefits of outdoor play that were intrinsic to our childhood experiences and an in-depth exploration of the reasons behind the potential lack of these experiences for today's children:

1. Physical Health

- Then: Outdoor play is a vital part of childhood development, involving many physical activities like running, jumping, climbing, and playing sports. These activities actively enhance children's muscle strength, endurance, agility, and overall physical coordination. Simultaneously, outdoor play serves as an effective means for children to expend energy, aiding in the promotion of a healthy and active lifestyle.

- Now: In today's fast-paced world, many children are adopting sedentary lifestyles, largely due to the pervasive presence of screens, extended hours spent playing video games, and tightly packed schedules. This shift toward a more inactive way of life is resulting in decreased levels of physical activity among children, which in turn can lead to a range of potential health issues, including but not limited to obesity.

2. Creativity and Imagination

- Then: Immersing oneself in the natural world, whether through hiking in the forest, climbing trees, constructing elaborate forts, or engaging in imaginative play, plays a significant role in nurturing creative thinking and problem-solving skills in children. When children are given the freedom to explore unstructured environments, they are able to invent their own games, establish rules, and let their imaginations run wild, fostering a sense of creativity and ingenuity.

- Now: Children may find their creativity hindered by predefined rules and limitations in environments with structured indoor play and digital entertainment. These settings may provide fewer opportunities for children to freely engage their imagination and allow their thoughts to flow without constraints.

3. Social Skills and Emotional Development

- Then: Participating in outdoor group activities such as team sports, outdoor games, and group challenges provided opportunities for children to learn how to communicate effectively, navigate conflicts, and collaborate with others to achieve common goals. These experiences fostered teamwork and cooperation and contributed to the development of emotional intelligence, resilience, and interpersonal skills, which are essential for their social and emotional well-being.

- Now: Due to the growing trend of children engaging in indoor activities, whether alone or in virtual environments, the opportunities for them to enhance their social skills through direct face-to-face interactions have been greatly reduced. This shift in behaviour has significant implications for developing social competencies among children.

4. Connection to Nature and Mental Well-being

- Then: Engaging in outdoor activities such as hiking, birdwatching, or camping allows us to immerse ourselves in the natural environment, fostering a profound sense of connection to the world around us. This connection, in turn, has been found to significantly reduce stress levels and contribute to a more peaceful and balanced state of mind. For children, in particular, exposure to nature has been shown to help them develop emotional regulation skills, promoting mindfulness and a better understanding of their own emotions

- Now: In today's fast-paced world, many children have limited opportunities to experience nature's wonders, which can adversely affect their mental and emotional health. With more time spent indoors, they may feel confined and miss out on the benefits of outdoor exploration. Additionally, frequent exposure to screens can contribute to heightened overstimulation, further impacting their well-being.

Reasons for Reduced Outdoor Play

- Safety concerns: Parents may have concerns about safety, which could lead them to restrict outdoor activities for their children.

- Urbanisation: In contemporary urban areas, the absence of

ample green spaces and playgrounds may limit children's opportunities to engage in outdoor exploration and play, potentially hindering their physical and cognitive development.

- Technology addiction: Children are increasingly involved in digital entertainment, including activities such as playing video games, using tablets, watching TV, and using smartphones.

- Busy schedules: The combination of challenging academic responsibilities and the diverse array of extracurricular engagements leaves very little room for unstructured free play, leading to a scarcity of leisure time.

Encouraging Outdoor Play Today

- Create Opportunities: Encourage outdoor play by taking your children to local parks where they can run, play, and explore nature. You can also plan family outdoor activities such as hiking, biking, or picnicking in the park. Additionally, allow your children to have unstructured playtime in the backyard or at a nearby playground where they can use their imagination and creativity to engage in free play

- Limit Screen Time: Set specific time limits for screen usage and allow designated periods of the day for outdoor activities. This will help create a balance between digital and physical activities, promoting a healthier lifestyle.

- Foster a Safe Environment: Find safe and accessible

outdoor areas where children can play freely.

Encouraging children to engage in outdoor play can have numerous benefits for their physical, mental, and emotional development. Just as many of us experienced in our own childhoods, the opportunity for unstructured play in natural environments is crucial for a child's overall well-being. It's important that a child learns to be self-sufficient and adaptable regardless of the situation, season, culture, environment, location, or the people they are surrounded by. Every aspect of a child's surroundings plays a role in their development, and outdoor play is essential to their growth.

Suggested Routine for a Family:

- **4:00–6:00 AM**: Wake-up time for the family.

- **6:00 –8:00 AM**: Breakfast together or individually before heading to school or work.

- **12:00–2:00 PM**: Lunch, either packed for school/work or eaten together at home.

- **6:00 – 8:00 PM**: Dinner as a family, followed by light conversation or relaxation.

- **7:00 – 9:00 PM**: Wind down time—limit screens, read, or enjoy family bonding activities.

- **9:00 – 10:00 PM**: Bedtime routine for children, with parents following shortly after.

By implementing various effective strategies and finding the right balance between structure and flexibility, families can successfully overcome the common challenges associated with waking early, going to bed on time, maintaining daily routines, and effectively managing weekends and holidays. These efforts can lead to healthier habits, reduced stress levels, and a more harmonious and fulfilling family life.

SUMMARY

Establishing a structured family routine is vital for the well-being of all members, yet it comes with several challenges. Key issues include the difficulties of waking up early, maintaining consistent sleep schedules, coordinating mealtimes, adhering to daily routines, and managing changes during weekends and holidays. These challenges can increase stress and unhealthy habits if not effectively addressed. Strategies for overcoming these challenges involve creating a consistent sleep schedule, fostering positive morning routines, planning regular mealtimes, organising daily tasks, and maintaining structure during weekends and holidays. Engaging in shared activities like gardening can also enhance family bonds. Ultimately, a disciplined routine nurtures healthier habits, reduces stress, and cultivates a harmonious family environment, allowing for personal growth and stronger connections. By prioritising these practices, families can embrace a fulfilling lifestyle anchored in well-being and togetherness.

06(B)

Minimalism:
A Lifestyle of Purpose

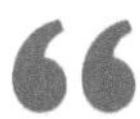

"Minimalism is the art of letting go so that life's true essentials have space to shine."

Minimalism is more than just a trend; it's a conscious lifestyle choice that focuses on simplicity, intentionality, and reducing excess to make room for what truly matters. In a world overflowing with distractions and material possessions, minimalism encourages us to declutter our lives—physically, mentally, and emotionally—and focus on the essentials. By embracing this lifestyle, we allow ourselves to strip away the unnecessary and cultivate a sense of clarity, balance, and contentment. Minimalism isn't about deprivation but rather about enhancing well-being by removing clutter that doesn't contribute to our goals or values. Through intentional living, one can experience reduced stress, increased fulfilment, and a deeper appreciation for life's simple pleasures.

Embracing Minimalism in Daily Life: Aligning Physical, Mental, and Emotional Aspects

Adopting minimalism as part of your daily routine impacts more than just the physical space around you. Minimalism aligns your physical, mental, and emotional well-being, bringing harmony and balance to every facet of life. Here's how:

1. **Physical Simplification**: Minimalism begins with

decluttering your physical surroundings. A clean, organised space is visually calming and makes it easier to focus and be productive. Start by removing unnecessary possessions, paring down to only what you need and love. This reduction of material excess encourages a simpler, more functional environment, allowing your space to breathe. You'll find that a clutter-free environment brings clarity and prevents the overwhelming feeling that often comes with excess. This physical alignment creates a foundation for mental and emotional clarity.

2. **Mental Clarity**: Minimalism extends beyond your environment—it is also about decluttering your mind. We're constantly bombarded with information, decisions, and distractions that can overwhelm us. Minimalism encourages you to streamline your tasks and focus only on what is essential, reducing mental noise. By prioritising fewer activities and cutting out what's non-essential, you free up mental energy for creativity, problem-solving, and reflection. Morning routines, for example, can be simplified to involve only meaningful tasks that set a positive tone for the day [As outlined in the earlier sections of this book]. By focusing on essentials, you make decisions with greater clarity, avoid burnout, and experience more peace of mind.

3. **Emotional Balance**: On an emotional level, minimalism helps foster a sense of calm and contentment. By stripping away excess and avoiding emotional clutter,

such as toxic relationships, unnecessary worries, or unresolved conflicts, you cultivate emotional resilience. Minimalism teaches acceptance and contentment with what you have rather than constantly seeking more. By engaging in mindful practices like gratitude and letting go of perfectionism, you foster emotional stability and joy in the present moment. Simplifying your life emotionally helps reduce anxiety, stress, and emotional fatigue, leading to a greater sense of emotional balance and fulfilment.

Daily Routine: Integrating Minimalism for Holistic Well-Being

To truly embrace minimalism and align your physical, mental, and emotional aspects, integrate it into your daily routine from morning until night. Much of what is introduced in this chapter has already been touched upon in earlier parts of the book. Here, it serves as a brief reflection, tying everything together from a minimalist perspective.

1. **Morning Simplicity**: Start your day by waking up early in a clutter-free environment. A minimalist morning routine might include simple, purposeful activities such as stretching or yoga, journaling, or a few moments of quiet reflection. Avoid unnecessary digital distractions and focus on the essentials that set a positive tone for the day. Physical alignment begins with a tidy space, mental clarity with a focused mind, and emotional balance with calm and gratitude.

2. **Intentional Focus Throughout the Day**: Simplify your to-do list by focusing on just a few critical tasks rather than overwhelming yourself with too many. This promotes mental clarity and ensures that your efforts are spent on meaningful activities. Make sure to take mental breaks and engage in physical activities that nourish your body, like walking, exercising, practising breathing techniques or simply being in nature. This holistic approach nurtures your body and mind while maintaining emotional equilibrium through balanced, intentional living.

3. **Mindful Eating and Fasting**: Adopting minimalist practices around food can also align physical, mental, and emotional health. Intermittent fasting, for example, encourages mindful eating, allowing your body to detox and function at its best. This simple, intentional approach to nourishment reduces decision fatigue and emotional stress around food. Choosing simple, healthy meals instead of overindulging in excess sustenance promotes better physical and emotional balance.

4. **Emotional Detox and Relationships**: Simplifying your relationships is equally important. Focus on quality over quantity when it comes to social interactions. Maintain meaningful connections with loved ones and avoid unnecessary social commitments that drain you emotionally. This helps align your emotional well-being with the principles of minimalism. By letting go of toxic relationships and valuing those that truly matter, you

create space for joy and emotional stability.

5. **Evening Wind-Down**: As the day comes to an end, practice a minimalist evening routine to help you unwind and prepare for restful sleep. Engage in calming activities such as reading, journaling, or practising gratitude. Eliminate screen time or excessive stimulation that can disturb your mental peace. A minimalist wind-down routine helps your mind relax and emotionally centres you, leading to better sleep and overall well-being.

Conclusion: A Holistic Minimalist Life

Adopting minimalism as a lifestyle choice integrates the physical, mental, and emotional aspects of your daily life. By decluttering your physical surroundings, streamlining your thoughts, and fostering emotional balance, you create a space that allows you to focus on what truly matters. Minimalism not only reduces stress but also enhances your overall well-being by aligning your priorities with a simple, intentional life. From waking up early in a clutter-free environment to winding down with a peaceful evening routine, minimalism can help you live a more fulfilling, balanced, and meaningful life, one that prioritises joy, purpose, and contentment.

ENDNOTE
Rise Early, Thrive Daily!

As we conclude our journey into the art of **Rising Early**, let us take a moment to appreciate the profound influence that a disciplined routine can have on our lives. Rising early bestows upon us precious moments of tranquillity, allowing us to set our intentions and cultivate a lifestyle rich in well-being. The shared nutritious meals, the laughter echoing around our dining tables, and the mindful moments spent together weave a vibrant tapestry of connection and fulfilment, nourishing both our bodies and spirits.

In the words of Todd Stocker, *"A sunrise is God's way of saying, 'Let's start again.'"* Each daybreak symbolises a fresh opportunity to reset our minds, renew our spirits, and reorient ourselves toward our goals. Embracing the rhythm of early mornings opens the door to the boundless potential each day holds. These sacred hours grant us the gift of self-reflection, personal growth, and the nurturing of our most cherished relationships. In the stillness before the world awakens, we discover clarity in our thoughts and intentions, setting a positive tone that resonates throughout the day.

Early mornings become a time to connect with ourselves, fostering harmony among our minds, bodies, and emotions. Within this serene space, we can engage in practices that honour our unique aspirations—whether it's expressing gratitude, practising mindfulness, enjoying gentle movement, and most of the other enriching habits discussed in this book. Each of these activities serves as a stepping stone toward a more fulfilling life. By weaving these practices into our early routine, we create a powerful momentum that carries us through daily challenges, illuminating our paths with purpose and intention.

In this beautiful journey, we come to realise that **Rising Early** transcends mere routine; it is a heartfelt commitment to ourselves and our families. It forms the foundation of a vibrant, purpose-driven life where well-being thrives, and each day is approached with renewed energy and optimism. As we prioritise our health, we inspire those around us to embark on their own journeys of intentional living.

Let us cherish the invaluable lessons learned and the transformative practices embraced. In the embrace of dawn, we uncover not just a new day but a fresh start—an opportunity to live fully, love deeply, and thrive together. Each morning invites us to release yesterday's burdens and step into a realm of endless possibilities. With every sunrise, we are reminded of our resilience, our strength to move forward, and our power to shape the lives we desire.

Join us on this journey illuminated by ***"The Magic of Rising Early,"*** Let each daybreak guide you toward a more meaningful and enriched life. Let's celebrate the beauty of ***rising early*** and the profound transformations it inspires, weaving a vibrant tapestry of joy, connection, and fulfilment into our everyday lives.